Achieving Success Through Community Leadership

Achieving Success Through Community Leadership

Peter A. Weil, Richard J. Bogue, and Reed L. Morton

Health Administration Press
Chicago, Illinois

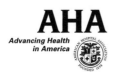

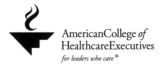

Your board staff or clients may benefit from this book's insight. For more information on quantity discounts, contact the Health Administration Press Marketing Manager at (312) 424-9470.

05 04 03 02 01   5 4 3 2 1

Library of Congress Cataloging-in-Publication Data

Weil, Peter A., 1945–
    Achieving success through community leadership / Peter A. Weil, Richard J. Bogue, and Reed L. Morton.
        p. cm.
    Includes bibliographical references.
    ISBN 1-56793-166-9 (alk. paper)
        1. Community health services.   2. Leadership.   I. Bogue, Richard J.   II. Morton, Reed L., 1944–   III. Title.
    RA427 .W454 2001
    362.1'2—dc21

                                                2001039917

The paper used in this publication meets the minimum requirements of American National Standard for Information Sciences—Permanence of Paper for Printed Library Materials, ANSI Z39.48-1984. (TM)

Project manager: Helen-Joy Bechtle; Cover/text design: Matt Avery

Health Administration Press
A division of the Foundation
    of the American College
    of Healthcare Executives
1 North Franklin Street
Suite 1700
Chicago, IL 60606-3491
(312) 424-2800

American Hospital Association
1 North Franklin Street
28th Floor
Chicago, IL 60606-3421
(312) 422-3000

Contents

Figures

Preface

This book is about helping hospitals relate to their communities. It identifies practices that the authors uncovered in visits to hospitals that were slightly ahead of the curve in providing for their communities' health needs. By studying and documenting what the hospitals' leaders were doing to improve their communities' health, we focused on processes that ideally could be employed by any hospital seeking to gain or regain its legitimacy.

Why should a hospital adopt the practices described in this book? For one thing, not-for-profit status is contingent on the hospital's provision of healthcare to the community. Certainly, the hospital cannot provide for all the health needs, but not-for-profits derive their legitimacy and social support from the perception that they are working to meet community needs. Leaders must at least try to care for the community's needs—that is, the needs as defined by the community.

In addition, the hospital staff's commitment to the hospital may be affected by the institution's commitment to meeting the needs of the community. While studies have shown that financial remuneration is one factor in helping organizations recruit and retain valued employees, studies have also found that employees want to feel that they are part of a worthwhile endeavor that serves a useful societal function. For example, a recent study of the major sources of job satisfaction of certified nurse assistants showed that they are motivated primarily by the joy and fulfillment they find in taking care of people. External factors, namely pay and other incentives, ranked second on the motivational scale (Robertshaw 1999).

By linking the organization's goals to community health needs, the hospital will increase the long-term commitment of employees and medical staff. Leadership has a responsibility to build a culture that honors the hospital's goal to improve community health.

Because leadership about community health is so important and so visible to the community, proactive measures can ensure that the hospital does not get mired in the day-to-day problems of financial solvency and proving that quality services are provided. These are valid concerns of the hospital but not to the exclusion of the mission and vision of providing healthcare to the community.

By "community," we are referring to a geographically circumscribed area in which residents are likely to use the hospital's services. Some hospitals define community a little differently. For example, some hospitals serve a particular religious group or fraternal organization (e.g., Masons) or people with special illnesses (e.g., rehabilitation hospitals). Any of these groups could be considered a hospital's community.

THE NOTION OF PRACTICES

When we began this study—and throughout our travels—nearly all of those we interviewed wanted to tell us about the good things they were doing for and with their communities. We had to stop nearly everyone at least once—and some more often—to remind them that for this study we were not interested in what was being done to intervene against a specific problem in the community but in changes in the organizational culture. Many others have created and communicated lists of community interventions; we were focused on the rituals and habits of hospitals intent on sticking to their community health mission.

A "practice" is a routine behavior that can be described well enough so that someone else can understand what it would be like to adopt that behavior. To move toward the goal of financial success, hospital boards and managers engage in many practices for monitoring and adjusting performance. For example, financial reports are produced and reported frequently. External audits are conducted, reviewed, and approved on a regular basis. Similarly, annual strategic planning retreats and marketing plans ensure that the hospital provides needed services to its customers.

Practices also describe how hospital leaders strive toward the goal of quality: accreditation standards are reviewed and met, and accreditation visits are prepared for and hosted; medical audits are conducted regularly; and peer review occurs on an ongoing basis through specific methods. Continuous quality improvement initiatives, benchmarking, and critical pathways are all practices designed to ensure the hospital provides high-quality care. And personnel practices help hospitals keep up with contemporary employee benefits such as employee opinion surveys, salary surveys, health and retirement plans, as well as vacation, sick leave, and paid-time-off policies.

All these practices are part of a routine set of activities that define and describe how a hospital acts to get one or another part of its work done. Taken together, they make up what goes on in a hospital. In other words, they describe the behaviors that both create and give information about the organization's culture.

But no commonly recognized practices exist to ensure that hospitals hold themselves accountable to serve their community. The goal of this project was to document the practices hospitals conduct to ensure attention to community health. We aim to help hospitals and health systems shift their cultures toward community health through the adoption of new routine practices.

The operative concept is that small steps begin a journey. Every hospital can begin to discover or rediscover its community health purpose by adopting some of the practices outlined in chapters 1 through 7. In the introduction we discuss how we uncovered leading practices and how we tested these on a group of demonstration sites. We also provide a brief overview of how to use this manual and what other resources are available to you and your leadership team as you consider implementing some of these practices. Chapters 1 through 7 define and describe the leading practices we hope you will consider adopting. We conclude with a "lessons learned" chapter 8, as well as sources for continuing your learning on this topic.

REFERENCE

Robertshaw, N. 1999. "Understanding the Needs of Direct Care Staff." *Provider* 10 (Oct. 25): 39–53.

In everyone's life at some time our inner fire goes out. It is then burst into flame by an encounter with another human being. We should all be thankful for those people who rekindle the inner spirit.

—Albert Schweitzer, M.D.

Acknowledgments

We want to thank the leadership teams that welcomed us and taught us about their hospital management and governance practices: Cambridge Health Alliance, Cambridge, Massachusetts; Camcare, Inc., Charleston, West Virginia; Citrus Valley Health Partners, Covina, California; Crozer-Keystone Health System, Springfield, Pennsylvania; Memorial Healthcare System, Hollywood, Florida; Memorial Hospital and Health System, South Bend, Indiana; Mission Hospital Regional Medical Center, Mission Viejo, California; Evergreen Community Health Care, Kirkland, Washington; Kaleida Health, Buffalo, New York; Maria Parham Hospital, Henderson, North Carolina; St. Joseph Healthcare, Albuquerque, New Mexico; St. Mary Medical Center, Hobart, Indiana; Texas Health Resources, Irving, Texas.

We owe a great debt to our National Advisory Panel who guided our selection of leading and demonstration sites, and evaluated our interviews and our final products including a casebook that is located on ache.org, our video products, and this book. They exercised the right balance between pushing for quality and meeting deadlines! The panelists were: Paul K. Halverson, Dr.P.H., FACHE, (chairman), director, National Public Health Performance Standards Program, Centers for Disease Control and Prevention, Atlanta, Georgia; Jameson A. Baxter, president, Baxter Associates, Inc., Palatine, Illinois; Errol L. Biggs, Ph.D., FACHE, director, Center for Health Administration, University of Colorado, Denver; Douglas D. Hawthorne, FACHE, president/CEO, Texas Health Resources, Irving, Texas; F. Rob Johnson, manager, Health and Welfare Plans, Eastman Chemical Co., Kingsport, Tennessee; Carolyn Lewis, Washington, DC; Jane Oehm, Golden, Colorado; Bruce D. Peterson, FACHE, administrator, Mercer County Hospital, Aledo, Illinois; Malvise Scott, vice president, Programs and Planning, National Association of Community Health Centers, Washington, DC; Bernard Turnock, M.D., clinical professor, School of Public Health,

University of Illinois at Chicago, Chicago, Illinois; and Bruce Vladeck, Ph.D., professor of health policy, Mt. Sinai Medical Center, New York. Thanks too, to our external evaluator, Suzanne Miel-Uken, director of health policy, Public Sector Consultants, Inc., Lansing, Michigan.

Staff of the American College of Healthcare Executives and the American Hospital Association deserve our thanks especially for the care that they took to scrutinize our writing and the time our supervisors allowed us (far more than we anticipated) to accomplish our task. Rita Harmata, Ph.D., CHE, deserves special note for her willingness to assist the study team on their site visit to St. Joseph Healthcare. We appreciate especially the staff of Health Administration Press—notably Helen-Joy Bechtle, for her careful reading and editing of this manuscript.

Finally, we want to thank Robert DeVries, LFACHE, and Terry L. Wright of the W. K. Kellogg Foundation for their support of this project. We began this project believing that it would be sufficient to study how CEOs and boards were evaluated as the key to motivating community health. Our project evolved into something much more comprehensive. We appreciate the latitude the Foundation gave us to study the wide array of practices that promote community health in hospitals.

Introduction

INCREASING CONCERNS ABOUT THE HOSPITAL'S ROLE IN COMMUNITY HEALTH

After the implementation of the prospective payment system in 1984, hospitals were encouraged to behave more like businesses. Patients that were admitted to a hospital in the Medicare program were to be covered for their costs based on their illness. This fixed rate of payment changed the way hospitals conducted their work. Suddenly, restricting the use of resources in caring for patients became beneficial, since a flat fee would be paid for any given diagnosis. The era of plentiful resources and unrestricted care for the insured came to a close.

Some hospitals abused the new system, urging physicians to discharge patients too soon or coding patients' illnesses as more serious than they were. Other hospitals, feeling the new emphasis on financial matters, engaged in expensive competition for doctors' loyalty, adopted a predatory posture, or developed lines of business that detracted from the overall benefit delivered to the local community. Most hospital leadership teams began developing a "strictly business" culture, designing most decisions around the "bottom line" of the organization's financial position. Thus the new system, although originally intended to stem the rising costs of hospital care, fostered a shift in hospital culture that raised the stakes on financial performance while often pulling attention away from other forms of excellence.

Before long, many people outside hospitals learned that hospitals' leaders were speaking and acting in ways that indicated they valued financial matters higher than other concerns. Community activists, newspapers, attorneys general, judges, and local politicians began to challenge the prioritization of values among hospitals. Not-for-profit hospitals in particular were called to task. In 1985, Utah challenged Intermountain Health Care to show that it provided community benefit. The challenge was triggered by allegations that the health system had refused care to an uninsured patient. IRS rules state that to retain their deemed status as not-for-profit corporations, not-for-profit hospitals must operate free of private inurement and deliver an overall benefit to the community as a whole. This could be argued to mean delivering certain levels of charity care, participation in universally available government programs such as Medicare, or delivering emergency services to anyone who requires them (Gray 1992, 10).

By the late 1980s, a number of state attorneys general were challenging the notion that not-for-profit hospitals should remain tax exempt. In response, two well-known community health activist-scholars published an article on what not-for-profit hospitals should be expected to do in return for their tax exemption. J. David Seay and Robert Sigmond, in "Community Benefit Standards for Hospitals: Perceptions and Performance," argued that five distinguishing features define the voluntary hospital (Seay and Sigmond 1989):

1. Community values
2. Governance and accountability
3. Institutional mission and relationship with physicians
4. Long-term commitment to the community
5. Provision of a locus and focus for voluntarism and volunteering.

They argued further that all of these features should be evident in a hospital's mission statement. This book will illustrate how these issues permeate the efforts of leading hospitals today.

On the first feature, community values, Seay and Sigmond stated that

There are many aspects of healthcare services delivery, including hospital services, that cannot be accounted for or fully understood by means of an economic transactional analysis alone. Also there are numerous healthcare services that communities often value and want to have, regardless of the government's willingness to provide them or their ability to be profitable enough to interest commercial entrepreneurs (p. 11).

Thus, hospitals are somehow set apart from the free market economy and government—producing services like rehabilitation and obstetrical services that are not fully reimbursed but are nevertheless considered important and represent what the community values in healthcare.

The second feature that distinguishes the voluntary institution pertains to governance and accountability—was the institution created to profit investors, to function as a governmental entity, or for some other end? Trustees in hospitals have sworn allegiance to the hospital above the opportunity for personal gain and have promised to continually assess the environment in setting policies.

Hospital-physician relationships are represented by the third feature distinguishing the community hospital. Such hospitals must be more than simply doctors' workshops; instead, leaders must try to address what they perceive to be unmet community needs.

Fourth, the institution's commitment to the community must be long term. Instead of being strictly market driven, it must respond to market demand but also remember that demand is not a complete measure of the entire community's healthcare needs. In essence, leaders of hospitals—trustees and executives—cannot give up trying to be creative in providing for the needs of the entire community in the face of adverse financial circumstances.

Volunteering and voluntarism is the fifth feature that characterizes community hospitals—they should be places where public-spirited individuals can "express themselves by giving of their time, energies, and funds in support of a special cause or institution" (Seay and Sigmond 1989, 14).

Seay and Sigmond also suggest community-oriented hospitals routinely evaluate their success in achieving their goals. This, of course, includes having set goals (often in the form of mission statements), determining if processes are in place to conduct such an examination, and demonstrating outcomes that show community health involvement.

For example, hospitals might investigate the governance structure and accountability relationships by asking, "Are physicians, members of the community, and patients involved in the governance and operation of the hospital?" The hospital might study how much charity care is provided or whether a policy is in place that states that patients will be cared for regardless of their ability to pay. Other outcomes to measure might include whether the hospital addresses the unmet needs of the community as demonstrated through mortality, morbidity, and health status statistics. Planning initiatives summarized in a community benefit plan could help define the community hospital's outcomes.

These features represent the principles that define the community-oriented hospital. Seay and Sigmond also suggest that the Joint Commission on Accreditation of Healthcare Organizations create a community benefit standard to define and measure the extent to which hospitals are adhering to these principles. Key practices that Seay and Sigmond recommend include partnering with other community organizations that "can provide input with respect to the community's health problems and practical approaches to dealing with these issues" (p. 26). Importantly, public health departments are among the most significant links for hospitals, and the authors decry the "costly separation of environmental health initiatives, other public health initiatives involving healthy living habits, and the initiatives of the medical and hospital establishment."

Seay and Sigmund also present recommendations about the functioning of a community benefit hospital's structural elements—that is, the board, medical staff, and management. For example, the board must appoint individuals who are concerned with the health status of the community. The CEO should be evaluated, in part, on commitment to the hospital's community benefit goals and ability to work effectively in the community. Reports on the progress of achieving community goals should routinely be received by the board. In not-for-profit hospitals, medical staff bylaws require that staff members ensure that all patients in the service area receive cost-effective, quality care. Management is to provide leadership in responding to the health and other human service needs of the community.

In the discussion of specific practices that comprise the main body of this book, many of these features of the hospitals are portrayed. The main difference between Seay and Sigmond's initiative and ours is that they believe a national accrediting agency should be set up to ensure that community hospitals adhere to these principles. We, on the other hand, prefer a more bottom-up approach—and suggest that hospitals begin to take on practices that promote community benefit but do so voluntarily and according to what they perceive they can handle at the moment. David Jeppson (1989), in responding to the Seay and Sigmond manifesto, suggested that not-for-profit hospitals'

> . . . primary tool is our mission in word and deed. We must communicate and demonstrate our mission whenever we have the chance, and we must create new opportunities to do so. We must be prepared to articulate our mission and set high goals to reach community service needs (p. 43).

NATIONAL INITIATIVES TO PROMOTE COMMUNITY BENEFIT

In the past decade and a half, a number of national initiatives have promoted the provision of community services by not-for-profit hospitals (see Table I-1).

HOSPITALS' CURRENT IMAGE PROBLEMS

Although the national initiatives gave useful guidance to hospitals, studies did not demonstrate an improvement in the public's perception of hospitals. Indeed, in 1999, the AHA issued a video depicting ordinary Americans describing hospitals as mercenary organizations that had largely abandoned their caring missions. Even today, healthcare executives have indicated a desire to know more about building a positive image in the community (ACHE 2000).

In a recent interview on how hated firms should handle being disliked, Leonard Schaeffer, CEO of Wellpoint Health Networks, stated,

The most important thing is not to be defensive. You have to try to understand the concerns of customers and key constituents and take corrective action. You have to do things companies in other industries do, then you have to try harder to be a better listener and be more responsible inside and outside the company. Companies must take a leadership role within an unpopular industry to solve problems.

You have to have a clear and elevating goal. You have to be in business for a reason that inspires employees. We are in a business that helps our customers get the healthcare services they need. There is a big tension around cost, but the goal is meaningful and inspiring. (Shaeffer 2001)

Mission and Employee Retention

Mission statements set out the organization's philosophy and priorities. In theory at least, one of the primary purposes of mission statements is to realize better staff motivation/management control toward achieving a common organizational purpose or "sense of mission." Mission statements begin a process of providing employees with a meaning for their work that transcends the immediate needs of their department or even the organization (Henry and Henry 1999). Unfortunately, however, little empirical research exists to confirm or refute this (Bart and Baetz 1998). A few studies in the general management literature show that goals positively influence employee commitment (Barrick, Mount, and Strauss 1993; Wright et al. 1993).

Turnover of clinical staff is a major issue facing hospitals and other healthcare organizations. Part of the turnover problem may be caused by inadequate efforts by organizations to orient their employees, especially with respect to the mission of the organization. In their comprehensive analysis of turnover, Ulschak and SnowAntle (1993) conclude,

In the final analysis, the most compelling reasons nurses enter nursing and stay in it are still the original ones. The fulfillment of helping others maintain or regain health or die peacefully is as much at the heart of nursing as it has ever been (p. 153).

A recent survey of certified nurse assistants, who provide 80 to 90 percent of personal care to residents of nursing homes, showed that they are motivated in their work primarily by the joy and fulfillment they find in taking care of people. This intrinsic source of satisfaction ranked higher than such extrinsic motives as compensation and various forms of recognition (Will and Simmons 1999).

Today, Florida cites a shortage of more than 10,000 nurses, and Minneapolis–St. Paul reports a 10-percent nursing staff vacancy rate for all healthcare organizations (Coile 2001). Many other categories of health workers are also in short supply (e.g., radiation technologists and pharmacists). According to a futures study (Coile 2001), labor shortages will get worse and bonuses and recruitment incentives will not solve the issue. Coile concludes, "no easy solutions to labor shortages are in the pipeline."

Coile's strategic advice is for executives to work toward retention, not recruitment, as the most cost-effective strategy available to hospitals. Specifically, executives should make their hospital a "magnet hospital" that focuses on staff satisfaction (Coile 2001). In our view, the ultimate magnet effect occurs when staff believes that the hospital is carrying out its mission to work toward improving the community's health.

This project comes at a time when hospitals face a considerable image problem relative to their contribution to their communities and key shortages of personnel. These issues are solvable, and our search for solutions included interviewing leading hospitals that are regarded as major contributors to their communities' health and as good places to work. We think that by sharing the practices they use to accomplish these outcomes, you can accomplish similar effects in your hospital.

METHOD OF RESEARCH

For the purposes of our study, "leading" hospitals are those that have the most experience and have adopted the most sophisticated techniques for linking performance expectations to community health. To develop the list of potential leading case sites, we pursued a multistaged process. First, we reviewed the published literature. Second, we retrieved data from recent surveys conducted by both ACHE and AHA about CEO pay-for-performance practices and governance evaluation mechanisms. Third, we asked for input from sister organizations such as the Catholic Health Association, Healthcare Forum, VHA Inc., Western Consortium for Public Health, and various state and metropolitan hospital associations. These efforts yielded a list of about 50 potential leading sites.

To narrow the 50 potential sites to a more manageable list, we developed a fax survey that contained eight questions that we thought represented "core practices" relative to management and governance performance tied to community health. The questions were as follows:

(1) Are report cards issued on the hospital's performance to the community?
(2) Are executive salaries or bonuses tied to community health indicators?
(3) Does the CEO's job description reference community health?
(4) Does the board have job descriptions that include a focus on community health?

(5) Does the board conduct a self-evaluation that includes a focus on community health?

(6) Are board members selected with community health issues in mind?

(7) Are data on community health used in board meetings?

(8) Are data on community health used in the written strategic plan?

We received responses from about half of those surveyed. Some CEOs said they did not belong on the list of leading sites, but many that did respond said that they had incorporated some of the eight items about which we inquired.

We then took the results of this fax survey to our national advisory panel. The panel suggested that we interview 17 CEOs about the above questions in greater detail. After conducting those interviews, we reported the results and made our recommendations to the national panel. The panel agreed with our selection and we notified the hospital CEOs of their selection as "leading sites." Selected were:

1. Cambridge Health Alliance, Cambridge, Massachusetts
2. Camcare, Inc., Charleston, West Virginia
3. Citrus Valley Health Partners, Covina, California
4. Crozer-Keystone Health System, Springfield, Pennsylvania
5. Memorial Hospital and Health System, South Bend, Indiana
6. Memorial Healthcare System, Hollywood, Florida
7. Mission Hospital Regional Medical Center, Mission Viejo, California

Each of these seven leading practice hospitals or health systems hosted a two-day site visit during the summer and fall of 1999. The purpose of these site visits was to identify, explore, and document specific management and governance practices that establish and implement individual and organizational performance expectations in the area of community health.

Each site visit consisted of a series of interviews with between 10 and 14 individuals. Interviews were conducted with informants identified in advance of the site visits as filling certain key roles in the organization or the community. Informants included the CEO, the current board chair, the board secretary, the senior vice president or chief operating officer, the medical staff president, the head of fundraising or the foundation, and the vice president with responsibility for community health programming. We also interviewed the executives of two or three community organizations involved in community health partnerships with the hospital or health system and others based on the initiatives and corporate structure of the leading practice sites.

Eight interview protocols were designed, each reflecting the likely areas of knowledge for each kind of informant. However, all interviews were designed around the following basic structure:

(a) A review of the specific practices discussed in the fax survey and subsequent telephone interview that link performance expectations to community health, as well as any new practices uncovered at this site. This helped define the study's boundaries and obtain new information about these practices.

(b) A review of the informant's responsibilities and exploration of the informant's observations about any other specific practices that might be used in the organization.

(c) Solicitation of new information to strengthen the interviewers' evolving understanding about those specific practices that had been discovered in previous interviews or during this interview.

As the two-day visits progressed, an overall pattern of discovery emerged. Earlier interviews typically identified new practices. By the end of the first day, or early in the second day, during step (a) of the interviews the informants usually confirmed the set of practices that had been identified and rarely identified new practices. Therefore, interviews that were conducted later in the visit usually concentrated much more attention on step (c), exploring and confirming details about the new practices that had been identified.

In all cases, a final debriefing interview was conducted with the CEO. In addition to reviewing what had been learned, the interviewers asked for further description of any specific points that remained unclear and for a list of documents pertinent to the practices that had been identified. These procedures resulted in 25 specific management and governance practices for linking performance expectations in hospitals and health systems to community health.

Selecting and Working with Demonstration Site Hospitals

A project that attempts to disseminate various practices from leading hospitals to others has to examine how transportable these practices are in new venues. Therefore, we sent out a call for proposals to all community hospitals in the United States to apply to become a "demonstration site." The project's National Advisory Panel helped staff select six hospitals. The staff chose hospitals for their expressed interest in adopting leading practices, but also took into account diversity in geography, size, system membership, and other variables. Selected were:

1. Evergreen Community Health Care in Kirkland, Washington;
2. Kaleida Health in Buffalo, New York;
3. Maria Parham Hospital in Henderson, North Carolina;
4. St. Joseph Healthcare in Albuquerque, New Mexico;
5. St. Mary Medical Center in Hobart, Indiana; and
6. Texas Health Resources in Irving Texas.

The complete background and experiences of the demonstration sites are documented in our casebook located at www.ache.org.

HOW TO USE THIS BOOK

This book identifies 25 different practices that a hospital can use to advance its community health mission. The list of practices is presented as Figure I-1. The practices are categorized by seven unique strategies. By considering each of the seven strategies defined below, decide on the strategy that seems most appropriate for your initial efforts. Then, once the strategy is chosen, focus on the practices within that strategy. Each of the strategies constitutes a chapter in this book, and within each chapter we include associated practices for the strategy.

DEFINITIONS OF THE SEVEN STRATEGIES FOR LINKING PERFORMANCE EXPECTATIONS TO COMMUNITY HEALTH

1. Visioning a Healthy Community

The board and management can use the organization's vision and mission statement, operational goals, and evaluation of organizational goal achievement to emphasize community health as an expectation for performance throughout the organization. Practices that accomplish visioning community health show the organization's employees and communities that boards and executives take seriously their organization's role in community health because they widely communicate the vision and regularly assess performance against the vision.

2. Financing to Promote Community Health

Simply talking or writing about helping improve the community's health is not enough. Hospitals can successfully establish a systematic and sustained financial commitment to community health, eliminating the risk of coming

Figure I-1: Leading Practices to Motivate Community Health

A. Visioning a Healthy Community
   1. Instill values about community health through goals
   2. View consolidation or merger as an opportunity to evaluate mission
   3. Evaluate multiple bottom lines

B. Financing to Promote Community Health
   4. Invest in community health systematically
   5. Compensate management

C. Educating About a Healthy Community
   6. Invest in education
   7. Establish a curriculum that incorporates community health

D. Personnel Decisions to Foster Community Health
   8. Establish a senior management position for community health
   9. Integrate the evaluation of the CEO, board, and organization
   10. Encourage staff involvement in other community organizations
   11. Have a stable, long-tenured executive team
   12. Expand the role of the hospital CEO to include management of public health

E. Marketing Activities that Enhance Community Health
   13. Collect community health information
   14. Issue report cards
   15. Multi-brand—to promote community health with and through partners
   16. Connect to consumers through information systems
   17. Hold recognition events to honor community health activists

F. Creating Structures that Institutionalize Attention to Community Health
   18. Create a community health information unit—especially through public/private partnerships
   19. Develop an Institute for Community Health
   20. Establish a committee of the board to promote quality and community health
   21. Include staff on board committees
   22. Develop and work strong support networks within the community

G. Developing Processes that Promote Community Health
   23. Conduct CEO calendar audits of community health activities
   24. Have an ongoing board improvement process
   25. Channel marketing costs of competitors to benefit the community

up short during lean years and demonstrating to leadership that financing community health can mean improved performance for the organization too. To effect such sustained commitment, it may be advisable to tie executive compensation to community health objectives. Investing in community health in this way allows hospitals to walk the talk.

3. Educating About a Healthy Community

Educating about community health provides boards and executives as well as staff and community members with the knowledge base for understanding community health as an important part of what the hospital does. Methods of education are many—ranging from teaching boards about the determinants of health, to developing a regular program for educating managers and new employees about the hospital's vision and values and what it does to further community health objectives. These educational practices help to put awareness of the community on par with the clinical, financial, and regulatory and legal contexts of the hospital's provision of healthcare.

4. Personnel Decisions to Foster Community Health

Personnel decisions for a health community include creating a senior management position that reports directly to the CEO and is responsible for community health programming, community partnerships, and outreach issues. Other practices include encouraging the CEO to become involved with public health issues, using community health criteria in CEO and board evaluations, and encouraging staff to become involved in other community organizations. Long tenure of executives appears to promote trust among the leadership team and innovation in meeting the community mission.

5. Marketing Activities that Enhance Community Health

Although commonly viewed as a way to generate more business, marketing community health can make a lot of sense too. Marketing research methods can help hospitals identify and understand health assets and issues in the community. Hospitals can generate positive outcomes for the community and themselves by marketing community health rather than just the organization or its services. By distributing reports to the community, hospitals send a reminder that they are wellness organizations, and not only a place to visit when sick; the hospital can also report on whether goals are being achieved. Leading hospitals partner with other community organizations and sponsor recognition events to honor community health activists.

6. Creating Structures that Institutionalize Attention to Community Health

Several organizational arrangements can promote the community health enterprise. By creating a formally organized unit of the hospital to promote some element of community health, managers can institutionalize the hospital's involvement in community care rather than rely on the commitment of single individuals. Two examples of structures created within hospitals to advance the public's understanding of the level of community health achieved are a health information unit or a special health institute. Other structures include establishing foundations or specialized councils that help to involve community members and raise funds to support outreach efforts.

7. Developing Processes that Promote Community Health

Some practices link performance expectations to community health through ongoing processes that do not fit easily into the other six practice areas. These processes reflect a continuous service improvement perspective. For example, to ensure the CEO attends to the organization's community health agenda as much as the financial or clinical quality agendas, a periodic calendar audit could be conducted. Or, the board might consider obtaining at the end of each of its meetings third-party feedback about how well the board attends to community health matters and elicits the views of all members.

In addition to this book, two sources of information are available to help you implement these strategies into practice. The first is the videotape that accompanies this book. Titled *Rekindling the Flame: Achieving Success Through Community Leadership*, it is available for purchase by calling 301/362-6905. The second source of information is located in the research publications area of our web site, www.ache.org. The casebook presented there provides rich detail about all of the leading practices that we discovered in each of the seven leading sites. A complete description of the experiences of the six demonstration site hospitals in trying to implement one or more leading practice is also included. Finally, we urge you to contribute to our message board on www.ache.org in the "Affiliates Only" area to relate your own experience in establishing one or more leading practice. (Nonaffiliates of ACHE can log onto the message board with "Guest" as the ID number and "Kellogg" as the last name.)

REFERENCES

American College of Healthcare Executives. 2000. "Affiliate Needs Survey." Chicago: ACHE. [Unpublished study.]

Barrick, M. R., M. K. Mount, and J. P. Strauss. 1993. "Conscientiousness and Performance of Sales Representatives: Test of the Mediating Effects of Goal Setting." *Journal of Applied Psychology* 78 (5): 715–22.

Bart, C. K., and M. C. Baetz. 1998. "The Relationship Between Mission Statements and Firm Performance: An Exploratory Study. *Journal of Management Studies* 35:6 (Nov.): 823–53.

Coile, R. C. 2001. *Futurescan 2001: A Millennium Forecast of Healthcare Trends 2001–2005.* Chicago: Health Administration Press.

Gray, B. H. 1992. "Why Nonprofits? Hospitals and the Future of American Health Care." *Frontiers of Health Services Management* 8 (4): 3–32.

Henry, L. G., and J. D. Henry. 1999. *Reclaiming Soul in Health Care: Practical Strategies for Revitalizing Providers of Care.* Chicago: Health Forum Inc.

Jeppson, D. H. 1989. "A Time for Action by Not-for-Profit Hospitals." *Frontiers of Health Services Management* 5 (3): 40–43.

Omenn, G. S. 1999. "Caring for the Community: The Role of Partnerships." *Academic Medicine* 74 (7): 782–89.

Seay, J. D., and R. M. Sigmond. 1989. "Community Benefit Standards for Hospitals: Perceptions and Performance." *Frontiers of Health Services Management* 5 (3): 3–39.

Schaeffer, L. 2001. "Interview: Hated Firms Have to Try Harder, Avoid Defensiveness." *USA Today* Jan. 1: 6B.

Ulschak, F. L., and S. M. SnowAntle. 1993. *Managing Employee Turnover: A Guide for Healthcare Executives.* Chicago: American Hospital Publishing, Inc.

Will, K., and J. Simmons. 1999. "Ohio CNAs Speak Out." *Provider* 10 (Oct. 25): 107–10.

Wright, P. M., J. George, S. R. Farnsworth, and G. C. McMahan. 1993. "Productivity and Extra-role Behavior: The Effects of Goals and Incentives on Spontaneous Helping." *Journal of Applied Psychology* 78 (3): 374–81.

CHAPTER ONE

Visioning a Healthy Community

B LOODY MARY IN the famous Broadway musical, *South Pacific*, said it best, "If you ain't got no dream, then how you gonna make a dream come true?" The board and management create mission and vision statements as well as goals to provide direction to the hospital. In doing so, they can emphasize community health as an expectation for performance throughout the organization. When leaders identify community health as a key objective and communicate this to staff and community members, the stage is set to pursue the other strategies that promote community health.

INSTILLING VALUES ABOUT COMMUNITY HEALTH THROUGH GOALS

Management science has made great strides in healthcare over the past decade. More and more healthcare organizations are adopting performance management systems that tie organizational strategy upward to vision and mission and downward to individuals' performance goals and objectives. Typically, financial and to a somewhat lesser extent clinical performance goals make up the concrete, measurable core of these performance management systems. Some organizations, however, are discovering new synergies and making better strategic decisions by embedding population and community health goals in the performance management system.

Cambridge Health Alliance

The business plan of the Cambridge Health Alliance in Cambridge, Massachusetts, is directly tied to community health outcomes. For example, an Agenda for Children was developed in Cambridge that was the product of a city-wide effort. The effort involves 25 elected officials plus parents and other community leaders representing 45 community agencies.

Multiple ongoing efforts had been in effect that related to improving the lives of children, some of which were duplicative and with little or no coordination between the efforts. The Agenda for Children, with involvement of the Kids Council, School Department, Human Services, and the Alliance, was established to coordinate the activities and set city-wide priorities. After several meetings, the group decided on two major initiatives for the short term: first, that all children should be able to read by the third grade, and second, that there be an adequate supply of quality, supervised preschool and after-school activities. Because in many households both parents work, the after-school activities were a special concern for children aged 11 to 14. Interestingly, access to healthcare ranked eighth out of nine programs considered by the council, a commentary on the health systems' success in this area.

One key structural factor that allows Cambridge to effect community health initiatives is the fact that all chiefs of services are full-time employees and 185 physicians are employed by the system. This number includes not only all of the primary care physicians, but also all surgeons, emergency room physicians, anesthesiologists, and pathologists.

Another example of tying business planning to community health involved the possible closing of the obstetrics department, where 500 deliveries occurred per year resulting in a loss of $1.2 million annually. To respond to the community's preference for easy access to obstetrical services, Cambridge heard the pleas of staff and the community and established a nurse midwifery program. The nurse midwifery program is more cost effective than the traditional obstetrical care.

A final example concerns the financial arrangements by which public health is provided in Cambridge. Through a seven-year contract with the city, Cambridge Health Alliance provides a vast array of public health services for annual city support totaling $7.5 million. Tying public health activities with the services of an integrated delivery system has thus far served the community by attempting to ensure coordination of preventive, curative, restorative, and palliative care.

Memorial Healthcare System

The leaders of Memorial Healthcare System in Hollywood, Florida, advise that strategic plans serve a community health perspective better when they are less focused on a set of specific community health status measures. They prefer instead to use a broad array of health and quality of life information. Memorial's use of community quality of life data for direction setting and performance monitoring started through United Way's Compass methodology. MHS contracted with David Smith, of Smith Abt, to conduct a Community Health Needs Analysis. Frank Sacco, the CEO, serves currently as the chair of the Coordinating Council of Broward. Data from the health component of the survey were considered and nine initiatives were submitted to the MHS board for their consideration. The board, representing various geographic areas (and population segments) MHS serves prioritized these nine to focus on seven areas. These initiatives became the basis for MHS's strategic initiatives. The areas of focus included

1. Physician development
2. Quality improvement
3. Community commitment
4. Financial and operational viability
5. Organizational development
6. Customer focus
7. Market development

The initiatives have broadened over time. For example, initially the focus was on South Broward County, which is MHS's primary service area. Likewise, at first the board considered only adult healthcare services, but eventually added children's healthcare to the list of goals. Indeed, in the most recent strategic plan, health goals have been expanded to include more general, quality of life issues—today, children's and seniors' services are part of MHS's agenda, as is cultural diversity.

Attracting light industry to the service area to provide better paying jobs has been a major thrust of the initiative. In this case, Mr. Duncanson, the current board chairman, pushed for this initiative. Other community health efforts are spearheaded by the community health subcommittee of the board.

Mission Hospital Regional Medical Center

Mission Hospital Regional Medical Center in Mission Viejo, California, has developed a one-page summary sheet providing at a glance their mission, values, vision, and goals (Figure 1-1). Such deliberate integration of vision and goals allows the system to keep its core purpose at the forefront.

CONDUCTING A GAP ANALYSIS TO RECRUIT PARTNERS

A process used by several CEOs that serves to promote links to partners is for the CEO to conduct a gap analysis. Such analysis requires that the

MISSION
(Why We Exist)

To extend the Catholic healthcare ministry of the Sisters of St. Joseph of Orange, by continually improving the health and quality of life of people in the communities we serve.

VALUES
(What We Believe In)

Dignity
Excellence
Service
Justice

VISION
(What We Are Striving to Become in Next 5 Years)

To be recognized as a leader in providing regional integrated healthcare, promoting health improvement, and creating healthy communities.

STRATEGIC GOALS
(Major Initiatives Over Next 3–5 Years)

1. Collaborate with the community to identify, understand and respond to community needs impacting health and quality of life.

2. Achieve seamless, holistic (body, mind, and spirit), patient-centered care across the continuum through the integration of regional delivery systems.

3. Foster a work environment that attracts, retains, and develops values-based employees, physicians, and volunteers.

4. Build and sustain strategic partnerships with physicians and other providers that are value-based.

5. Uniformly measure and continuously improve clinical and service quality.

6. Proactively advocate for just public policy, and increase access to care.

7. Manage costs and allocate resources for effective stewardship.

FY 1999 STRATEGIC GOALS
(Major Initiatives Over Next 3 Years)

1. **Healthy Communities**–Develop community relationships and implement collaborative planning efforts to improve health and quality of life.

2. **Integration/Seamlessness of Regional Delivery System**–Develop a specific plan for enhancement of seamless, holistic (body, mind, spirit), patient-centered care across the continuum and begin implementation.

3. **Human Resources**–Foster a work environment that attracts, retains, and develops values-based employees, physicians, and volunteers.

4. **Physician Partnership and Integration**–Increase the number of affiliated physicians and enrollees in integrated relationships. Support and strengthen existing integrated physician partnerships through values integration, leadership development, enhanced communication, and operations improvement.

5. **Clinical Quality/Service Improvement**–Implement processes to track and improve clinical quality, as measured by the system-wide common clinical indicators. Share best practices and implement systems/processes to improve patient satisfaction and service.

6. **Advocacy**–Implement system-wide and entity-specific advocacy action plans to address system and local priorities, ensuring focus on children (access to care, food/nutrition, welfare reform).

7. **Stewardship**–Achieve budgeted financial performance for FY99, ensuring a balance between short- and long-term financial and strategic priorities. Understand and prepare for future initiatives requiring significant financial investment.

8. **Managing Growth**–Effectively plan for the Medical Center's growth.

CEO or other leader develop a vision of what community health should be relative to what it currently is. Such analyses can be based on data, or they can emerge from the leader's own views of underlying factors that contribute to community health.

Camcare, Inc.

Phillip Goodwin, CEO of Camcare, Inc. in Charleston, West Virginia, considers that Camcare's job is to identify health needs to be met and then see that something happens to fill the gap in service. The means of improvement is integral to Mr. Goodwin's vision for Camcare. Camcare approaches a group or individual that might have an investment in the issues associated with the gap, and then aids that group in taking ownership for meeting those needs. Camcare has been an incubator for a significant number of community-related entities that now stand on their own. Among these are West Virginia Health Right, Ronald McDonald House, a progressive nursing home (Hodges Center), and the Kanawaha Coalition for Community Health Improvement.

LESSONS FROM THE DEMONSTRATION SITES

Kaleida Health

Kaleida Health in Buffalo, New York, elevated community health and wellness to top-level goals in the strategic plan. Kaleida began a partnership with the local Catholic health system, and under the aegis of the United Way, held a community health Summit for the eight-county area. The Summit was not Kaleida's event, instead the United Way was slated as the lead organization and the local D'Youville College helped organize it. Thus, while initiated and supported by Kaleida, the Summit was conducted so that all the partnering organizations received equal billing. Rural groups in particular felt welcomed by the choice of the easily accessible fairgrounds as the site for the Summit.

Facilitating the Summit's reaching its objectives were: (1) early advertising; (2) holding planning meetings to help spread the word; (3) using the United Way as the lead agency; (4) obtaining the assistance of D'Youville College; and (5) keeping a low budget. Barriers to the event were: (1) keeping the invitation mailing in-house—it should have been outsourced, and (2) not resolving early on how exactly the collaboration would take place.

Prior to the demonstration site visit, the organization had three community initiatives incorporated in their strategic plan; after the Summit they identified seven. Each initiative is a reportable item to the board and is included as an element in the incentive plan for designated managers.

St. Mary Medical Center

St. Mary Medical Center in Hobart, Indiana, planned to expand the role of the mayor's wellness council to become a community health council (CHC). The plan was to organize a community group to decide and work on the next project to make Hobart a healthier community. Members would be recruited from areas of the community including government, schools, churches, business, and so forth. The group would create its own vision.

Most of the individuals appointed to the CHC were CEOs; others had special expertise or interest in improving the Hobart population's quality of life. A special effort was made to include a spokesperson for the poor; for this reason the head of the local food pantry was recruited.

The first meeting of the CHC was scheduled to take place three weeks after our first visit. Factors that facilitated this CHC were that (1) SMMC had nurtured a good relationship with the mayor, (2) a facilitator attended informal meetings of non-SMMC organizations, (3) many of SMMC's senior staff were active in civic and charitable groups, (4) SMMC informed the mayor how the new council would advance the government's own goals, and (5) the mayor's sister worked as a nurse at SMMC. Barriers to establishing the CHC were: scheduling (it took weeks to convene the first meeting), and that a few individuals may have been appointed who work primarily as facilitators rather than doers, even though the CHC requires the latter.

Texas Health Resources

Texas Health Resources (THR) in Irving, Texas, developed guiding principles for community health (Figure 1-2). Their goal during the project year was to include community health as a regular item on the board agendas. Although this goal had not yet been achieved for all the local hospital boards, community health is a regular agenda item on the system board. Topics addressed include an overview of THR's philosophy, an update on the family violence prevention initiative, an update on the activities of the community health councils (local hospital leadership groups that report their perceptions of needed community services), and a year-end review. The update was easier to implement because it is presented as part of the committee reports and it is confined to 15 minutes.

Our work will be guided by the following principles:

1. We will be guided by our mission, vision, values, and faith traditions.
2. We will embrace a broad definition of health.
3. We will develop diverse, collaborative partnerships in multiple communities, with particular concern for the poor and underserved.
4. We will use the Community Health Improvement Process to define our initiatives.
   - We will conduct annual needs assessments and/or updates in each community served by a THS hospital.
   - We will respond to the voice of the community in choosing our initiatives.
   - We will serve as a resource broker, bridging community needs, resources, and assets.
   - We will be held accountable for our work through the development and identification of outcome measures.
5. We will respect and support local initiatives, while leveraging impact through one to three regional initiatives.
6. We will engage multiple stakeholders in community service:
   - employees
   - physicians
   - hospital volunteers
   - donors
   - attending clergy
   - community partners
7. We will strive to provide charity care and community benefit in excess of the government standard.
8. We will work with local administrators and physicians to develop an annual community benefit plan for each THS hospital and will provide a yearly accounting of our efforts to the Community Health and Benefit Policy Council, the Community Health Councils, the Boards of Governors and Trustees, and our communities.
9. We will consider an annual THR tithe.

THR also sought to incorporate community health goals into each local hospital's annual strategic plan. This was accomplished in all but one local hospital. However, achieving consistent results was difficult—some hospitals included goals that were very broad, others included clinical indicators even though the hospital administrators were taught how to conduct a community health improvement process. All hospitals had adopted the system-initiated, family violence prevention initiative at the time of our follow-up visit.

VIEWING CONSOLIDATION OR MERGER AS AN OPPORTUNITY TO EVALUATE MISSION

When hospitals merge and systems form, the challenges of managing the new entity become far more complex than before. With more sites and levels of care, more kinds of caregivers and layers of management, and more contracts and diverse cultures based on different missions, the leadership team needs rallying points to provide guidance to the staff, the physicians, the managers, and the board. The community health mission can be a powerful rallying point for the people at all sites and levels of today's increasingly complex healthcare organizations.

Crozer-Keystone Health System

The experience of Crozer-Keystone in Media, Pennsylvania, shows us that undergoing consolidation can represent an excellent opportunity to re-envision the organization and its purpose at the most fundamental level. The leadership and staff of the two merging hospitals needed a banner under which they could become one strong system, and the health of the community became a rallying point.

In Crozer-Keystone's case, successful consolidation meant figuring out how to deal with the values held by board members. As it happened, the board of one of the hospitals entering the merger had a strong and unshakable orientation toward mission, including the use of incentive compensation for top executives on the basis of some more general community service goals. The other board had focused its chief executive's evaluation almost exclusively on the hospital's financial performance. "The possibility of de-emphasizing mission in the resulting organization," said long-time trustee Robert Welsh, "was a non-starter." He thus inferred that the merger process could not begin if the mission was not agreed upon by the two parties. As a result of the mission-oriented board's insistence, the merger talks became infused with the question of how to ensure an emphasis on mission in the resulting organization. Incentive compensation on mission-oriented goals, as well as goals for finances and quality, became one method of solving this question.

Citrus Valley Health Partners

Merger created an opportunity to re-envision the role of Tom McGuiness, senior vice president for mission integration and community care, and to recharge the commitment to the community at Citrus Valley Health

Partners (CVHP) in Covina, California. The merger between Queen of the Valley Hospital and Intercommunity Medical Center in 1994 was a signal—and community health improvement provided a rallying point for the two cultures to merge.

Organizations should consider merger for both business reasons and for higher purposes. Indeed, at one point Mr. McGuiness suggested that organizations contemplate a shared mission to community first relative to mission—sharing that mission for a year or two, and only then, perhaps in the third year, considering merging the business of care delivery.

Kaleida Health

Kaleida Health is the product of two hospital systems and a children's hospital merging to provide healthcare for the community. Recently, Kaleida closed Columbus Hospital, Children's Hospital, and Millard Fillmore and combined them to build an $8 Million Family Medical Center. The merger was needed due to a downward spiral in available financial resources for the community's healthcare assets.

According to Bryant Prentice, Kaleida's first chairman, merger became possible because the chair and either the chair-elect or past chair from each of the merger entrants engaged in a series of meetings to discuss the reasons for the merger and the principles that would guide it. This "group of six" developed a set of merger principles, including establishing a steering committee whose actions required the approval of the board of each organization. This establishment of a set of guiding principles prior to entering formal merger discussions represents a leading practice, and also conforms to the AHA Board-approved Principles and Guidelines for Changes in Hospital Ownership and Control established in 1997. Figure 1-3 provides an example of the steering committee's merger evaluation principles for Kaleida Health. Such principles might guide an organization that is attempting to rally merging institutions around a community health mission.

EVALUATING MULTIPLE BOTTOM LINES

Related to the practice of instilling values about population and community health through goals is the idea of evaluating multiple bottom lines. Most managers think of the bottom line as the financial performance of the organization. But given a hospital's core functions as a clinical caregiver and as a major element of health provision in a community, creating a culture in which decision makers regularly evaluate multiple bottom lines can produce a more well-rounded and more sophisticated approach to strategic

FIGURE 1-3: EXAMPLE OF MERGER PRINCIPLES ENVISIONING
COMMUNITY HEALTH

1. The Buffalo General Health System, the Children's Hospital, and the Millard Fillmore Health System are committed to the community benefits that potentially could result from a merger of the three organizations into a new regional healthcare delivery system.

2. The governing board of each organization has the legal responsibility to study, evaluate, and reach its own conclusions regarding the potential merger and the unilateral right to withdraw from the merger evaluation process at any time prior to the execution of a definitive merger agreement, without prejudice, retribution, or financial penalty.

3. The steering committee shall establish the values, vision, mission, and guiding principles of Kaleida which will then require the specific approval of the board of each organization. We believe this activity must be of the highest priority in order to assess our commonality of understanding and compatibility.

4. The values, vision, mission, and guiding principles of Kaleida will serve as the foundation of Kaleida's overall policy and operational activities. It is the expectation that the administration of the study and evaluation process will be driven by the vision, mission, principles, and values of Kaleida.

5. The steering committee has the responsibility to coordinate and manage the merger study and evaluation process.

    A. The steering committee shall operate on a consensual basis. In the event a decision or action is reached by consensus but is identified as being in conflict with any organization, such a decision or action must be unanimous to become final or acted upon.

    B. The steering committee and the organizations are best served by the development of a merger study and evaluation plan as the first step. As such, the steering committee has endorsed the use of an active outside facilitation process using Merlin Olson of Deloitte & Touche throughout the study and evaluation stage.

    C. The study and evaluation stage will be completed on an expeditious basis but not later than February 1, 1997.

planning and decision making. One such bottom line measure should be community health improvement.

Citrus Valley Health Partners

Citrus Valley Health Partners CEO Pete Makowski stresses to the management team and the board that CVHP has multiple bottom lines:

There is the financial bottom line that is critically important because you can't go out and do these wonderful things and support these projects without the financial wherewithal. But also, the higher purpose is our mission that must be fulfilled.

John Izzo, in *Awakening Corporate Soul*, has been hired to work with Makowski and 14 individuals on the "mission core team." These individuals represent all areas of the hospital (primarily staff, not management). These individuals are the best ambassadors for the organization: they are upbeat, positive, caring, and compassionate, and they live the values of the organization.

With this team, Makowski hopes to identify the behaviors that CVHP performs well and those that it does not perform well. How are these behaviors measured? Tom McGuiness, the senior vice president for mission integration and community care serves as staff coordinator to the team and the mission officer is the CEO. Makowski now receives calls from around the country about organizational renewal; according to Makowski, healthcare providers are burned out because they are so focused on finances and affiliations. But attending to these objectives precludes the provision of good care.

McGuiness went to the Feltzer Institute and reports having a "sacred experience" on relationship-centered care. Makowski wanted his board to understand through a board retreat "the deep wisdom that exists within relationships," and to get in touch with their own individual deeper wisdom as well as their corporate wisdom as a board. The medical staff executive committee then requested a similar relationship-centered care retreat. This session was sponsored by the hospital and the medical staff cooperatively, and a small group of administrators and board members were present for the weekend retreat.

CVHP operates within a mature managed care market where the majority of patients are enrolled in managed care programs that are increasingly risk based. According to Armando Gonzalez, chair of the system board, it makes good business sense to try to enroll a healthy population. "A lot of people say our mission is to benefit the community. But the real truth is that in the future our margin will be *in* the community benefit." CVHP is seeking ways to show a pro forma financial benefit from the community benefit investments they make, fully expecting to find financial payoff for the organization from their intensive work to improve the health and quality of life of the communities they serve.

CHAPTER TWO

Financing to Promote Community Health

ONCE THE MISSION and vision of the hospital are translated into operational goals, boards and executives need to spend some time thinking about how to effect them. Allocating resources—financial resources, for example—to promote community health goals is a direct and measurable way to begin this process. In this chapter, we discuss how some leading hospitals tithe their net patient revenues so that community partnerships can grow. While tithing in times of adequate reimbursement can be in the form of money, tithing in lean years can sometimes take the form of allocating hours to help community partners. Apart from aiding partners, financial practices also include providing financial incentives for executives and staff members that meet or exceed community health objectives.

INVESTING IN COMMUNITY HEALTH SYSTEMATICALLY

Many hospitals and health systems dedicate specific amounts of resources to community health activities. In some cases, these investments take the form of a tithe, a percentage of margin that is set aside. In others, the investment may be made in public health activities that then restrains the growth of taxes in the community. Other systems make the investment in a specific target for charity care. Regardless of the method used, the key is a consistent, sustained, and systematic commitment to support community health. When financial support for community health is an important part of the organization's strategic direction, the organization can begin to shape itself in the interests of the community at large.

Memorial Hospital and Health System

Memorial Hospital and Health System in South Bend, Indiana, created a systematic approach to its community benefit activities by organizing them around a 10-percent tithe of its positive net margin. The approach *begins* with Memorial's strategic plan and its annual corporate goals and objectives.

Memorial's strategic goals are to:

1. Improve community health
2. Develop the integrated delivery system
3. Ensure the highest quality, services, and value
4. Improve quality of worklife

These four strategic goals, and the 10 to 15 specific and measurable objectives for each, are ubiquitous throughout Memorial. Staff and trustees refer to them frequently. They are widely used as touchstones for planning and for the evaluation of the performance of senior managers.

The tithing funds are used for the community health goals and objectives identified in the strategic plan, while the other three goals (develop the integrated delivery system; ensure the highest quality, services, and value; and improve quality of worklife) are funded through operations.

Proposals for community health projects are identified, reviewed, and refined through a community health action group (CHAG). CHAG is composed of seven to nine members who are chiefly members in senior management positions. The biweekly CHAG meetings are essentially open to any staff person, board member, or community leader who wishes to attend. At the time of our visit, CHAG was considering a request from a board member who wanted a regular seat in the action group.

CHAG works directly with partner organizations to identify and refine community health project ideas, and also decides which proposals are to be funded. One member of CHAG is appointed as champion for each evolving discussion and ongoing community health project. This relationship includes ongoing communication throughout the life of a project, which usually takes the form of biweekly meetings between a champion and each of the projects she or he champions. Any three members of CHAG can approve up to $10,000 in funding for a community health project. The process is intended to be organic and somewhat chaotic. No forms, deadlines, or any other "templates" have been established. The intent is to maximize the learning and innovation that can come from the tithing investments. The mental model is one of "collaborative learners"—not "check writers."

A committee of the board, the community health enhancement committee (CHE) reviews the strategic goals and objectives quarterly, and modifies them annually, as needed. In this context, the CHE receives quarterly information about progress in its various community health partnerships and projects. To select projects in which to invest, Memorial has developed a tithe-o-meter that allows the system to calculate the relative value of a partnership (Figure 2-1). The indicators included on this tool measure the ten characteristics deemed most important to the community. For example, Memorial's board uses the criterion of funding goal to consider whether a project's proponents expect it will become self-sufficient in the future. If so, the project is more likely to be endorsed and funded than if the project would require continuous funding from the hospital.

Chief operating officer Dan Neufelder identified one of the not-so-obvious benefits of strategic tithing. He noted that creating and managing the tithing process promotes dynamics for a community-health-focused management structure. More importantly, the tithing policy represents a means of encouraging community-health-oriented behavior by the entire organization in a way that demonstrates the true commitment of leadership. Staff are not expected to reduce investment in clinical services, for example, to invest in community health. Community health becomes instead another of the organization's core business practices with its own budget, complementing rather than competing with other important goals of the organization.

Mission Hospital Regional Medical Center

Mission Hospital Regional Medical Center in Mission Viejo, California, dedicates 10 percent of its net operating margin each year to Mission's social accountability budget. Seventy-five percent of this contribution is retained locally and is specifically allocated to care for the poor. The Camino Health Center consumes the bulk of these funds. The remainder is invested by the Community Benefit Committee of Mission Hospital in other priorities identified by Mission's community assessments. For example, Mission has recently funded:

1. The purchase of vans for senior transportation services;
2. The creation of a pediatric dental capacity in the Camino clinic;
3. The creation of a Family Resource Center (FRC); and
4. The contribution of a staff person to the FRC trained as a social worker who serves as FRC's executive director.

The other 25 percent of funds go to the St. Joseph's Health System Foundation. The largest allocation of these funds is to a disaster fund, which receives 75 percent of the system foundation's portion. Twenty percent of

Community Health Investment Value Scale

1. Partnerships Sought

□□■□□□□□□□□□□□□□□□□□□□□□□□
Few   Many

2. Target Population

■□□□□□□□□□□□□□□□□□□□□□□□□□
General   Underserved

3. Outcome Interest

■□□□□□□□□□□□□□□□□□□□□□□□□□
Short Term   Long Term

4. Investment Philosophy

■□□□□□□□□□□□□□□□□□□□□□□□□□
First Funder   Second Funder

5. Purpose of Funds

■□□□□□□□□□□□□□□□□□□□□□□□□□
Operations   Capital

6. Who We Fund

■□□□□□□□□□□□□□□□□□□□□□□□□□
Organizations   Individuals

7. Investment Objective

■□□□□□□□□□□□□□□□□□□□□□□□□□
Treatment   Disease Injury   Health
                        Prevention   Promotion

8. Investment Period

■□□□□□□□□□□□□□□□□□□□□□□□□□
1 Year   3 Years   5 Years

9. Funding Goals

■□□□□□□□□□□□□□□□□□□□□□□□□□
Continuous   Self-Sufficiency

10. Organizational Involvement

■□□□□□□□□□□□□□□□□□□□□□□□□□
Low   Medium   High

the system's portion is contributed to an endowment, which totaled about $12 million in 1998. Five percent of the system foundation's portion from the member hospitals is used for the Icon Award Program.

The endowment fund is intended as start-up or seed money for new investments in local communities. Member hospitals and others submit applications to the endowment fund seeking support for new efforts. For example, Mission Hospital submitted a request for support of an asthma education program for the schools. This asthma education program, which was funded by the endowment fund, relies on collaboration with the Saddleback Unified School District. As with other endowment-funded projects, staff is expected to find ways of making the asthma program self-sustainable. In this case, staff is communicating with insurers to encourage them to provide financial support for the full-time asthma educator in the schools.

In addition to the 10-percent tithe, 1.5 percent of operating costs are dedicated to healthy community initiatives. These efforts include education, cancer screening, smoking cessation, and other ongoing and more traditional efforts to promote health and well-being.

LESSONS LEARNED FROM DEMONSTRATION SITES

Evergreen Community Health Care

Evergreen Community Health Care in Kirkland, Washington, initiated a proposal process in which targeted subpopulations (elderly people who lack access to care, disabled elderly, and children with asthma) would submit a proposal and obtain a charter that provides businesslike rigor through careful project management. The team that evaluates the proposals uses a rating form so that evaluations would be standardized for all of those reviewed. One of the few barriers to this practice was that prior commitments had to be disengaged in a tactful and responsible way. Many of the prior grantees were given funds in smaller amounts for a couple of years so they could pursue other funding opportunities.

Texas Health Resources

Texas Health Resources in Irving, Texas, is planning to develop a strategy to systematically fund community health. They are reviewing desired benefits and outcomes in terms of both mission and margin; that is, they are making a business case for community health improvement as well as a mission case. They are also trying to link community health commitment to the organization's strategic direction. Finally, foundations are seeking sources of community support.

THR has allotted $2 million from foundations dedicated to community health. To derive a common definition of what constituted community health, interviews were conducted with all 14 local hospital presidents and others at the system level, as well as with leadership councils and physicians. A retreat for system council members was to be held to focus on the system's Family Violence Prevention Initiative and other policy matters. THR and Baylor, a former merger possibility, might collaborate on community health initiatives. Perhaps most interesting, a new system-level position has been created for community health evaluation to enable hospitals to see the benefit of their community health activities.

The senior vice president of corporate affairs at THR stated that she preferred to see community benefit integrated into the budget rather than allocated as a separate line item. The CEO expects each of the 14 hospitals to dedicate some funds to community health.

COMPENSATING MANAGEMENT

Incentive compensation systems are becoming increasingly common in healthcare. If some portion of the organization's strategy is concerned with community development and community health, then some portion of the incentive compensation system ought to be as well. This tight link between strategy and personal performance and pay can be a very effective and a regular reminder that the organization's strategy is not only to focus on financial viability and clinical quality but also on community health.

Crozer-Keystone Health System

Crozer-Keystone Health System in Media, Pennsylvania, has tied the bonuses of the CEO and 35 senior managers to the achievement of community health objectives. This came about because senior managers believe in the AHA and VHA mission of building healthier communities to regain public trust. Currently, hospitals are acting "too businesslike," and new partnerships need to be forged with community healthcare organizations.

To effect this reorientation, community health needed to be defined. To begin, Crozer-Keystone conducted experiments with local churches and invested in health programs there. Management convinced the board that linking bonuses to community health would be a sensible strategy.

Today, approximately 20 percent of the base compensation is a bonus opportunity for the 35 senior executives. Of their twelve to fifteen major goals, about one-third are related to the health status of the community. However, each executive must quantify his or her objectives unique to his or her area of responsibility. For example, Ed Baum, vice president for community health, has 50 percent of his objectives based on community health. In contrast, the vice president for the primary care network may have preventive goals for patients as a major part of his bonus potential.

This system has been in existence for four years. The system sets salary levels at the fiftieth percentile, but typically, with bonuses, individuals end up receiving remuneration at around the seventy-fifth percentile.

At issue now is how far down the organization such incentives should go. The system employs 6,000 people, and if the bonus system were to expand to include all of them, a decrease in base salary would of necessity result. The question is therefore how the four unions would react to such a change in compensation. In light of the bankruptcy of Allegheny, Mr. McMeekin, the CEO, feels he must be responsible in devising any changes to the compensation system.

Camcare, Inc.

The salary and bonus of all executives at Camcare, Inc. in Charleston, West Virginia, are tied to the four enduring strategic goals, including community health status improvement. Camcare's system of linking performance to pay is described as having three legs. The first leg is the use of surveys and an outside company to establish base pay at the fiftieth percentile for comparable organizations in other markets. Camcare evaluates all positions and specifically identifies outliers for more detailed analysis. All executive job descriptions have recently been reassessed.

The second leg is an incentive program that links 50 percent of the bonus of every executive from managers and up to system goals via individual goals that each manager helps to create for herself or himself. These bonuses are paid only when a positive margin occurs, which has occurred every year in the 1990s except for 1991 and 1998.

The third leg of linking performance to pay is a rich, three-tiered benefits program. The first tier is composed of the typical benefits. The executive, or second, tier typically includes an auto allowance, health club membership, financial planning services, will preparation, and association dues. The third tier is called ExecuFlex and emphasizes benefits that encourage stability, such as special life and disability insurance, similar special insurances for spouses, a capital accumulation plan, and a flex allowance plan that permits additional acquisition of investments. Approximately eight top executives also undergo performance and pay evaluation on the basis of explicit linkages with mission, plan, and annual goals for the system overall.

The chief executive's performance evaluation plan includes a 360-degree review. This review seeks input from all board members, the chiefs of staff,

Hospital/System	Who Is Eligible?	What Are the Basic Terms?
Crozer-Keystone Health Systems	CEO and about 35 senior managers	20% of base salary is bonus opportunity. About one-third of goals are community health goals.
Cambridge Health Alliance	CEO	20% of prior year's compensation is bonus opportunity. About 10% of effect is based on community health measures.
Citrus Valley Health Partners	CEO and all direct reports. All staff have a point system which translates into various symbolic rewards (tee shirts, cups, etc., and comp. time).	30% of base is bonus opportunity. 12.5% of effect for CEO is based on community health goals; varies for other managers depending on their areas of responsibility.
Mission Hospital Regional Medical Center	CEO, 9 direct reports, and 35 department managers	15% of CEO's compensation is community health related.
Camcare, Inc.	CEO and all executives	50% of bonus is tied to system goals, which include community health goals, and 50% of it is tied to individual goals.
Memorial Hospital and Health System	CEO and 15 senior executives. Examining how to tie compensation to community health for all staff.	50% of base is bonus opportunity. 13% of base is community health.

and direct reports. The CEO is rated on a four-point scale by each of these individuals, from whom comments are also solicited.

Table 2-1 presents a summary of the six incentive compensation plans that we encountered in this study.

CHAPTER THREE

*Educating About a
Healthy Community*

E DUCATING ABOUT COMMUNITY health can target as students the
hospital board, managers, staff members, and even community partners and members. Leading hospitals invest training funds so that their
boards are aware of national healthcare trends and best practices. They
also invest time and dollars to introduce their leaders to their community's
needs. This permits boards and key executives to make decisions that con-
form to the mission, vision, and goals of improving community health.
We found that leading hospitals systematically train their new employees
about the mission, vision, and goals the hospital is pursuing relative to
community health at the same time that they teach employees about the
patient care and the financial and quality objectives of the hospital.

INVESTING IN EDUCATION

Successful organizations in other industries are likely to invest in their
staffs. Healthcare organizations that dedicate a specific budget to education
around community health and the overall context in which the organization
operates are creating the capacity for future excellence. Such education and
information on the internal operations of the organization are extremely
valuable to the board, physicians, and staff.

Memorial Healthcare System

Memorial Healthcare System in Hollywood, Florida, makes a substantial
and regular investment in board member education. Each year all members
of the board and the chiefs of staff are invited to an Estes Park Institute
retreat in Naples. On a more frequent basis, board members' intensive work

with staff, as described under the topic of board committee structures in chapter 6, gives the board members a very high level of familiarity with issues faced by the organization.

Mission Hospital Regional Medical Center

Mission Hospital Regional Medical Center in Mission Viejo, California, invests generously in board education. All new board members undergo an orientation during which the Sisters of St. Joseph review their history and mission and the role of the congregation in governance. In addition, senior managers and members of the executive committee explain Mission Hospital's market and community context, its values and services, and board roles and expectations.

Board members regularly attend outside educational events, such as Estes Park's Institutes, and local opportunities conducted by institutions such as the University of California at Irvine. Edie Fee is a board member with a distinguished career and consulting practice as an asset manager for real estate and property management firms. She noted that, "The more I do for and with Mission Hospital, the more supportive management is of the need to provide me with educational opportunities." She added, "As we say in real estate, you cannot make the best and highest use of an asset unless you have been well educated to do so."

Mr. David Reed, chairman of the MHRMC board, freely admitted that as the former system CEO, he used to be a bit cynical about healthy communities. He had always been supportive of care for the indigent and other foci inside the hospital, but the idea of fixing a bend in the road to prevent auto accidents was a bit of a stretch for him at first. Through his education at Healthcare Forum's healthier communities program and through conducting a health assessment of the community, he became aware of population-based healthcare and began to recognize the necessity of focusing outside of the hospital limits to improve health in the community.

The Sisters of St. Joseph of Orange system, of which MHRMC is a part, conducts an annual trustee conference that focuses on governance responsibilities, roles, values, culture, and the system's goals and foci. The hospital also conducts an annual trustee conference that is attended by medical staff leaders and senior managers which emphasizes Mission Hospital's strategic issues.

The effect of a more intensive investment in board education is to enable board members to realize the values of the system and the hospital in their decision-making role. For example, in the 1997 flu epidemic, the hospital could have fit three patients in a room, with a positive benefit to its financial bottom line. However, this practice was rejected by the board in favor of offering the highest possible quality care to all its patients, reflecting the core value of "dignity." The patients who could not be accommodated were transferred to other hospitals.

Memorial Healthcare System

Memorial Healthcare System in Hollywood, Florida, has an executive with a community-wide scope of authority. John Benz, strategic business and development officer, dedicates 40 percent of his effort to oversight and leadership for staff in the following community-health-related areas: government relations, community benefit, community relations, marketing, and public relations.

A 1995 Fellow of the Healthcare Forum, Mr. Benz insists that his experience allowed him to meet with others who are committed to community health. These contacts are maintained virtually every day as he receives e-mails from colleagues who attended the Healthcare Forum Fellows Conference with him. He compares this fellowship to sharing a foxhole experience with other executives and counts on other members of that group to provide a support system on community issues.

Later when he, the CEO, and the system's board attended an Estes Park conference, Mr. Benz helped implement community outreach efforts. Such a protagonist is necessary, for as Mr. Benz suggested, "The CEO can't do it alone; he needs a co-chairperson to implement [the program] because the process is long and has hurdles [to overcome]."

This year MHS expects to invest in additional Fellowships as a means of developing the leadership skills of an additional senior manager and two local partners of MHS. MHS has also invested in special learning processes through Healthcare Forum, such as the Accelerated Community Transformation process.

LESSONS FROM DEMONSTRATION SITES

Evergreen Community Health Care

Evergreen Community Health Care in Kirkland, Washington, initiated a program for joint board, medical staff, and management education with instructors drawn from the local university. Key community leaders were also invited to attend. Scheduling difficulties were the only real barriers to effecting this practice, and the topics were selected by the CEO and the medical school dean. Polling of the leadership group on topics of interest may take place in the future.

ESTABLISHING A CURRICULUM THAT INCORPORATES COMMUNITY HEALTH

Some healthcare organizations have developed a regular program for orienting and educating staff about how the organization works, usually emphasizing budgeting and billing systems. Indeed, one of the leading practice sites has moved over 200 managers through an intensive eight-day course on the system, its context, its values, and how it operates. Building community awareness and community health into the regular management education programming of the organization can put environmental awareness on a par with near-term financial performance and can improve long-term strategy.

A COMPREHENSIVE APPROACH FOR MIXED TEAMS AND THE COMMUNITY

Memorial Hospital and Health System

Memorial Hospital and Health System in South Bend, Indiana, makes a substantial investment in the general education of trustees, staff, and community members. An important element of Memorial's education investment is its focus on trends and the environment in healthcare, rather than a focus on specific problems or issues. The goal of this investment is to increase the general capacity of the board, staff, and the community to understand and think strategically about healthcare and the system's long-term directions. In addition, Memorial arranges these educational experiences so that mixed teams of trustees, staff, and community leaders participate together in educational events as a way of increasing common understandings and shared vision. Involving mixed teams in educational programming also reduces barriers between staff and the board or other community leaders.

Much of this educational expense is paid for from the budget at the system level, rather than underwritten by department heads or individuals. Memorial easily spends over $100,000 per year on these educational activities which include packaged events like Health Forum's Best Practices Forums and governance programs of the Estes Park Institute, the Governance Institute, and others. In addition the system created its own annual Board Forums conducted in the Chicago area.

An especially valuable element of Memorial's education investment, according to many participants, is what Memorial terms its "Community Plunges." These plunges are theme-based learning experiences designed around site visits to address community health issues. These site visits bring mixed teams of people to neighborhoods, schools, congregations, and human services agencies, usually for several hours at a time, so that community leaders can gain a rich appreciation of the community's existing assets, the gaps in those assets, and the prospective role of each person to help improve the quality of life of the community.

Plunges reflect two key attitudes that seem to undergird Memorial's approach to community health. First, the leadership of Memorial assumes that adult learning should be experience based—as "hands-on" as possible. Second, the Memorial leadership assumes that participants start with little or no knowledge of the *real* determinants of community health problems. Instead, they seek to hear the stories of real people who live with and through these issues every day. Starting with few or no presumptions, these perspectives and stories consistently bring Memorial's leadership to some new clarifications of the best opportunities for investing in community health and well-being.

Jeff Gibney, executive director of South Bend Heritage Foundation, a community development corporation that is one of Memorial's local partners, put it this way: "Phil [Newbold, Memorial Hospital and Health System's CEO] is willing to admit his ignorance. He digs deep. He digs sincerely. And he is not condescending. If he were, we would not have a relationship."

Crozer-Keystone Health System

Crozer-Keystone Health System in Media, Pennsylvania, runs an ongoing staff education function called Crozer College. Crozer College gives 20 managers per semester a steeping in Crozer-Keystone culture and vision, as well as knowledge and skills for today's healthcare organization. Crozer College is composed of eight full-day sessions, delivered by members of the senior management team who teach components that are pertinent to their organizational roles. The participating managers are selected from throughout the organization on the basis of their past or likely future contributions to the organization's mission. As of the time of our visit, about 200 managers had gone through Crozer College. Figure 3-1 lists the fall 1998 curriculum for Crozer College.

FIGURE 3-1: EXAMPLE OF CROZER COLLEGE'S CURRICULUM

Tuesday, October 13

Welcome

Outline of program topics, logistics, expectations.
Participant project teams briefing. Background of Program, Vision, Mission, Goals, and directions ahead.

Thursday, October 29

Managed Care

Covers the tools that providers, such as Crozer-Keystone Health System, use to make informed decisions about risk-sharing arrangements with managed care organizations, insurers, and other payers. Provides a grounding in the general nature of risk associated with various payment mechanisms.

Linking Behavioral and Physical Healthcare

Exposes participants to innovative initiatives in different types of linkages by behavioral health providers, their benefits, and critical success stories.

Analyzing the Strategy for Maintaining a Healthy Community

Explains the how and why of developing partnerships between providers and community leaders to enhance the community's health status.

Monday, November 9

Transforming Healthcare Delivery

Explains the characteristics that community care networks have in common, the implications of these for an organization's mission, goals, culture, and governance, and the attitude shifts that underlie new delivery systems.

Creating an Environment for Innovation

Explores how to best foster a culture of innovation by focusing on key components such as goal setting, empowering, structuring, and funding.

Analyzing the Complexity of Human Resource Issues

Key strategies and issues for maximizing human resources, such as costs, benefits, staffing, development, and so forth, from a layman's point of view.

Friday, November 13

Team Project Development Day

Project teams meet to plan, finalize and prepare for final group presentations.

continued

The Legal Environment and Its Implications on Crozer-Keystone Health System

Overview of the predominant legal issues and litigation Crozer-Keystone is typically involved in and implications for corporate decision making.

Understanding Strategic Financial Decisions and Return on Investment

Through case study analysis, a question-and-answer examination of how and why strategic financial decisions are made from a corporate perspective.

Project Team Presentations

Individual team presentations. Project Team (#1 & #2 AM) – (#3 & #4 PM)

Graduation Reception at Springhaven Country Club 5:00 PM

CHAPTER FOUR

Personnel Decisions to Foster Community Health

P EOPLE ARE NECESSARY to translate a vision into reality. A number of practices were uncovered in our study that show how hospitals support their community health objectives by hiring, evaluating, and retaining key executives and staff who work to effect the community health vision. As in all sustained enterprises, leaders not only need to personally espouse the hospital's community health goals, but they should challenge others on the management team to get involved as well. We learned that some hospitals have effected their vision by recruiting and training a person they can trust—and one willing to take a few risks—to build partnerships with others in the community. Finally, we observed some interesting personnel practices that leading hospitals use to achieve the objectives of public health agencies in their communities.

ESTABLISHING A SENIOR MANAGEMENT POSITION FOR COMMUNITY HEALTH

The management teams of healthcare organizations have become increasingly professionalized and specialized. For clinical and financial matters, all except the smallest hospitals have specially trained staff reporting to the CEO. If population and community health is a key element of an organization's strategy, a senior manager with population and community health responsibilities seems a logical step for further improving the performance of healthcare organizations. Given their "extra-institutional" span of responsibility, senior managers of community health can be particularly effective in developing community partnerships, developing relationships with physician groups and other provider organizations, gathering objective market information, overseeing off-campus services, and identifying new opportunities for improvement.

Memorial Hospital and Health System

Memorial Hospital and Health System in South Bend, Indiana, has established a vice president–level position that serves as a community health intermediary, facilitator, and mediator with responsibilities at the national, state, and local levels. This position is based as much in the community as it is in the organization, reflecting the organization's broad approach to community health, including both social and economic issues in their definition of "health." A main function of this position is to identify health needs, resources, and potential partners. The current occupant of that role has a background in community development.

Citrus Valley Health Partners

As do other leading practice sites, Citrus Valley Health Partners in Covina, California, has a senior vice president overseeing community health efforts who reports directly to the CEO. In June of 1993, Tom McGuiness, senior vice president of mission integration and community care, relinquished half of his job, dropping oversight of several inpatient clinical and support department areas and human resources. He wrote his own job description to match the obligations expected for his new focus on community health. His responsibilities include overseeing organizational development and community care, but his concentration on each of these responsibilities has fluctuated. For the first four years, his job was 10-percent organizational development and 90-percent community care. Now, about 40 percent of his time is dedicated to organizational development. One of his specific duties is to spend about one-third of his time working with the Los Angeles County Department of Public Health on their system redesign process.

Throughout his tenure as senior VP of mission integration and community care, Mr. McGuiness has deliberately avoided building a bureaucracy inside the organization. While many senior managers define the scope and depth of their organizational power by citing the size of their budget or the number of FTEs they oversee, McGuiness rejects this as contrary to the interests of the organization and the community. Instead he aims to develop leaders and organizational capacities that will improve the health of the community. This does not necessarily translate into additional investment in partner organizations by the health system.

Memorial Healthcare System

Memorial Healthcare System in Hollywood, Florida, employs a similar strategic business and development officer, described in chapter 3. Figure 4-1 presents the job description that MHS has created for this position.

LESSONS FROM THE DEMONSTRATION SITES

Texas Health Resources

Texas Health Resources in Irving, Texas, hired a new executive vice president of corporate affairs to help focus the activities of both the Harris Foundation and the complementary Presbyterian Foundation relative to community health and benefit. This individual was expected to help determine which activities should be performed independently and which should be performed as a partnership. The foundations could not be integrated because each focused on different communities in various regions, and donors wanted to specify which communities their contributions would support.

INTEGRATING THE EVALUATION OF THE CEO, BOARD, AND ORGANIZATION

CEO evaluation practices in healthcare have become increasingly sophisticated. Organizational performance is becoming better understood as a combination of factors including clinical care, financial success, market share, customer and staff satisfaction, and community health outcomes. Regular board evaluations are expected under the standards of the Joint Commission for the Accreditation of Healthcare Organizations. Organizations exhibiting leading practices in performance evaluation link the CEO, board, and overall organization's evaluations consistently to mission, vision, and the strategic plan. They also include community health with the other major evaluation factors.

Memorial Healthcare System

Memorial Healthcare System in Hollywood, Florida, integrates CEO performance evaluation, board self-evaluation, and the board's evaluation of the organization's performance into a single annual cycle using the same

FIGURE 4-1: JOB DESCRIPTION OF STRATEGIC BUSINESS AND
DEVELOPMENT OFFICER, MEMORIAL HEALTHCARE SYSTEM

Reports directly to the Chief Executive Officer

Responsible for Government/Legislative/Regulatory Affairs
Responsible for Division of Strategic Business and Development

Direct Line Responsibility for the following areas:

Planning
    Strategic planning
    Program line development
    Grant writing
    Physician referral
    Patient transportation

Marketing and communications
    Overall communications program
    Marketing/advertising/production services
    MHS employee communications program
    Public/media relations
    E-commerce/Internet communications initiative

Community services
    Community First Initiative
    Coalition for a Healthy South Broward
    Community benefits/neighborhood empowerment programs
    Community relations
    Senior services
    KidCare Outreach

Community health services
    Primary care services
    School-based health services
    Children's Mobile Health Center
    Homeless health initiatives

Managed care services
    Managed care institutional modeling & contracting
    Physician contracting
    Credentialling
    Contract compliance
        Appeals unit
        Bad debt recovery unit
    Memorial Integrated Healthcare
        Uninsured patient fund
        Memorial managed care plan
        PHO/IPA administration
        South Florida community care network
        Disease and Demand management program

strategic initiatives and performance criteria. In March, Frank Sacco, the CEO, sends performance evaluation forms to the board members and to the system's four chiefs of staff. Both types of forms reflect MHS's strategic priorities and focus on the evaluator's satisfaction that each of a series of goals were well met, but the form used by the chiefs of staff is less detailed. Completed forms are returned and aggregated. The board chair and the CEO use this information in the review of the CEO's performance. The criteria used in this review include:

1. Fiscal management,
2. Community benefit and planning,
3. Peer review,
4. Quality improvement–risk management, and
5. Board and medical staff relationships.

Community-related performance comprises about 25 percent of total performance; this amount has grown over the past decade.

The CEO's salary increase is dependent on this review. The CEO's salary is pegged at a multiple of the staff's, and the chairman can increase it from 0 to 5 percent annually. (The full board could increase it more if requested.) No bonus is awarded to MHS's executives; the CEO has an executive employment contract.

In the early fall, the board conducts a special self-evaluation meeting. The same completed forms that had been used in the performance review of the CEO are used by the board members to assess and identify areas of improvement for their own performance and for the organization's performance. For example, if the board raises concerns about accounts receivable, it is likely that Mr. Sacco will be expected to address this issue both in terms of the board's education and in his own subsequent evaluation. Such congruency creates a reinforcing system that can focus the leaders' development in a short time span. The annual cycle of evaluation also includes a re-evaluation of the strategic initiatives and the performance review criteria.

Camcare, Inc.

Internally as well as externally, Philip Goodwin, the CEO of Camcare, Inc. in Charleston, West Virginia, is conscious that the changing healthcare market represents a lever by which to produce necessary and desired changes. Mr. Goodwin clearly accepts that care management in a continuum must ultimately predominate over the current episodic mode of treatment and payment, but recognizes that most people will not voluntarily abandon the rewards and security of the waning paradigm. The effective visionary leader must show the way and encourage those who are involved in the change.

The market can be a lever for change because it rewards those whose behavior aligns with its economic incentives. Corporate and governmental healthcare purchasers have become cost and quality conscious. They will contract selectively for high-value services even when the preferred vendor is no longer the local doctor or hospital. By demonstrating to the market that Camcare is improving health and producing superior outcomes, the organization begins to align with the evolving incentives of a market composed of prudent purchasers. Also, Camcare has established organizational and personal accountability for valued outcomes and has aligned its internal reward structure with achieving those outcomes. Figure 4-2 is the team assessment survey used by Camcare's executive team to help ensure personal accountability among team members.

FIGURE 4-2: TEAM ASSESSMENT SURVEY FOR CAMCARE, INC.
EXECUTIVE TEAM

Instructions: **Please provide a rating response (1–10) or don't know response for each of the statements listed below.**

Part I.

Scale									
1	2	3	4	5	6	7	8	9	10
Strong Disagreement		Moderate Disagreement				Moderate Agreement			Strong Agreement

This individual generally:

_____ 1. Treats people with respect and dignity.

_____ 2. Communicates openly and honestly with the team.

_____ 3. Role models the corporate values and management philosophy.

_____ 4. Appears to show respect for his/her peers.

_____ 5. Accepts responsibility for the customer-supplier relationships in which he/she interacts.

_____ 6. Is not overly protective of issues concerning his/her division/service group.

_____ 7. Is comfortable in a work environment where the need to "control" is de-emphasized.

_____ 8. Is able and willing to focus on both organizational goals and division/service group needs to ensure appropriate resource utilization and allocation decisions.

_____ 9. Is willing to discuss any issue the team wants to discuss (no "sacred cows").

_____ 10. Provides feedback to team members constructively, not negatively.

_____ 11. Shows respect for his/her subordinates.

_____ 12. Personally exhibits honesty and integrity.

_____ 13. Is not defensive in his/her reaction to feedback.

_____ 14. Tries to work toward mutually agreeable/win-win solutions to problems.

_____ 15. Appears to value education and development for himself/herself and fellow employees.

_____ 16. Is willing to express viewpoints that may differ from the group perspective.

_____ 17. Does not allow personality differences to affect working relationships.

_____ 18. Recognizes the value of employee satisfaction and employee relations.

_____ 19. Values diversity among the team.

_____ 20. Is able to disagree with team members respectfully.

_____ 21. Exhibits a positive attitude toward working with people.

_____ 22. Exhibits leadership characteristics consistent with continuous improvement philosophy and practice.

_____ 23. Creates and promotes a climate of trust in the team.

_____ 24. Recognizes team members for a job well done.

_____ 25. Demonstrates increasing understanding and commitment to the empowerment of subordinates.

_____ 26. Consistently tries to improve customer-supplier relationships with the team.

_____ 27. Appears to trust other members of the team.

_____ 28. Communicates with consideration of the needs of the receiver.

_____ 29. Gives credit to subordinates who deserve it.

_____ 30. Manages resources wisely and appropriately and with regard to organizational impact.

_____ 31. Supports team decisions.

_____ 32. Is adequately sensitive to diversity issues in the workforce.

_____ 33. Strives to continuously meet customer requirements in fact and in perception.

continued

FIGURE 4-2: CONTINUED

_____ 34. Is empathetic with the viewpoints of others in the team.

_____ 35. Demonstrates positive political skills in the organization.

_____ 36. Manages from the premise that employees are as important as financial goals.

_____ 37. Is forgiving of mistakes made by members of the team.

_____ 38. Provides well-timed communication and feedback to team members.

_____ 39. Effectively works with other areas to foster collaboration.

_____ 40. Professionally demonstrates high standards of ethical conduct.

_____ 41. Is willing to help other members in the team meet their goals.

_____ 42. Effectively and positively manages inter-divisional/service group conflict and removes barriers to organizational performance.

_____ 43. Does not appear to have hidden agendas when working with this team.

_____ 44. Supports education as an organizational goal/priority.

_____ 45. Addresses issues with other team members directly rather than behind closed doors/in cliques.

_____ 46. Attempts to understand and respect the needs of others (includes respondent) on the team.

_____ 47. Is personable and easy to approach with problems and issues.

_____ 48. Ensures alignment of organizational and divisional/service group goals.

_____ 49. Appears to role model the team process to subordinates.

_____ 50. Discourages perpetuation of rumors and false information.

_____ 51. Effectively aligns goals with other division/service groups.

_____ 52. Willingly accepts shared responsibility for the leadership of the organization.

_____ 53. Places organizational needs above divisional/service group needs.

_____ 54. Effectively communicates his/her position and feelings to the team.

_____ 55. Effectively keeps others informed of important goals, issues and developments within his/her division/service group.

_____ 56. Exhibits a high level of interest in working with this team.

_____ 57. Accepts ownership of team problems; does not assume issues are someone else's problem.

_____ 58. Demonstrates leadership characteristics worthy of organizational position.

_____ 59. Demonstrates a commitment to achieving team goals.

_____ 60. Openly encourages and accepts feedback from others.

_____ 61. Exerts a positive influence on team effectiveness and team relationships.

_____ 62. Resolves conflict in a timely manner.

_____ 63. Appears to personally enjoy other members of the team.

_____ 64. Is a team player.

_____ 65. Makes decisions in the best interests of our team's mission and goals.

_____ 66. Manages changes effectively.

_____ 67. Demonstrates an appropriate level of knowledge of the healthcare industry.

_____ 68. Makes effective and timely decisions.

_____ 69. Effectively communicates change to the team.

_____ 70. Remains current in his/her areas of expertise and responsibility.

_____ 71. Exhibits a willingness to make difficult or unpopular decisions.

_____ 72. Is flexible and open to change.

_____ 73. Exerts a positive influence on team decision making.

_____ 74. Accepts challenges to his/her ideas.

_____ 75. Demonstrates appropriate awareness of important issues facing Camcare.

_____ 76. Involves appropirate team members in change processes.

_____ 77. Demonstrates expertise in performing his/her role in the organization.

_____ 78. Involves appropriate team members in decisions that affect them.

_____ 79. Achieve his/her position/performance objectives.

_____ 80. Overall, is effective in performing his/her role.

Part II.

Instructions: **Remembering the purpose of this assessment process as individual growth and development, what is the single most important suggestion or recommendation for improvement that you could make to this individual. (Comments will be listed anonymously with all other comments.)**

Instrument development by: Ms. Sharon Hall, Camcare, Inc. and Dr. Michael Brookshire of Marshall University.

Cambridge Health Alliance

Apart from the compensation arrangements of the CEO, staff of Cambridge Health Alliance in Cambridge, Massachusetts, use a largely standard approach to performance evaluation. Senior staff write a self-assessment that is then reviewed and used as an improvement tool with their supervisors.

Although this process is not particularly unusual, it does drive a valuable set of leadership competencies into the organization as a result of the criteria that are used for this evaluation. These criteria include such leadership competencies as modeling collaboration, continuous quality improvement, and diversity leadership. While originally designed as part of the CEO performance evaluation, these leadership competencies have been introduced to senior and middle managers throughout the organization. Some of these other managers now make regular use of the leadership competencies in evaluating their own performance, as well as that of their staff. This process had not been highly formalized and had not entered all parts of the system at the time of our site visit.

LESSONS FROM THE DEMONSTRATION SITES

Evergreen Community Health Care

Evergreen Community Health Care in Kirkland, Washington, learned in its effort to incorporate performance objectives into the overall planning process that the board had to review performance objectives for the CEO in advance of the goals set for the hospital. By preparing the CEO's performance objectives early, the board's expectations can be solidified early in the year, which offers better, more consistent guidance to the CEO and his staff. In addition, management staff's performance expectations were enhanced specifically to emphasize that each team member is expected to be a community leader.

Kaleida Health

Kaleida Health in Buffalo, New York, revised its board's self-evaluation tool to include items such as bringing added value to the community and saving money. Similarly, management's proposed evaluation tool incorporates three major areas, one of which is mission-focused community service.

The 10-percent annual bonus opportunity requires managers to document various levels of contribution (including financial contributions) to organizations that are aligned with the mission of Kaleida Health. Voluntary service must be ongoing and applicable to the job held at Kaleida. Figure 4-3 presents the individual performance measurements developed by Kaleida Health.

Texas Health Resources

Texas Health Resources in Irving, Texas, has included a community health improvement imperative in its executives' performance evaluations. Community health improvement has become a core competency, and executives must document and prepare an action plan for individual key performance indicators. The competency has also been added to THR's 360-degree feedback evaluation and will become part of the directors' self-evaluations.

Differences were observed between the pre-merger systems (the Harris Methodist Health System and Presbyterian Healthcare Resources) in implementing these evaluations—particularly in how community health initiatives were measured. The CEO stated that the differences were included in overall performance measurements to ensure that everyone had knowledge of THR's objectives.

ENCOURAGING STAFF INVOLVEMENT IN OTHER COMMUNITY ORGANIZATIONS

A great way to build support and loyalty throughout the community is to have many active ambassadors for the healthcare organization. Encouraging staff to invest time in other community organizations can create a large, active sales force for the healthcare organization. Options for enabling this strong sales force include recognition and reward programs for employees. For example, consider granting reasonable and verifiable release time for this outside work or communicating widely about the staff's overall contribution as a result of the employer's encouragement of such voluntary efforts. Auxiliary benefits include enhanced staff morale, improved community awareness of challenges facing the organization, and additional suggestions for improving the organization's overall performance.

Memorial Healthcare System

Memorial Healthcare System in Hollywood, Florida, encourages its management and staff to volunteer in other community organizations. This

_____   _____
            Name   Job Title

The Annual Incentive Plan allocates 10 percent of the annual performance opportunity to recognize the importance of cultivating personal and professional growth and community service among the individuals who lead Kaleida Health. To be eligible for an incentive, the candidate must achieve at least a score of 1 in each of the 3 dimensions outlined. The amount of the incentive will be determined by computing the average of the top 2 of the 3 dimensions scored.

Summary of Score

	Self Score	Board Score
1. Personal and Professional Development		
2. Internal Leadership		
3. Community Service		

| Total of top 2 of 3 scores above | |
| Average of top 2 of 3 scores | |

1. Personal and Professional Development

A. List those educational and developmental activities, professional societies, and external committees that you actively participated in over the last calendar year. List your level of participation (i.e., office held, speaker, etc.)

I participated in the following:	Level of Participation	How did you apply these activities to your role at Kaleida Health?

B. Personal financial support of organizations promoting healthcare issues will be considered, if disclosed.

Organization Name	$$ Range of Personal Contribution	Location	Organizational Purpose

Scale: 0 = no evidence outside of required activities

1 = several examples of education activities, evidence of substantial active participation in professional organization.

3 = significant number of education activities that have impacted job performance, active involvement in professional organizations, committees, etc. Provides fiscal support.

5 = achievements as outlined in #3 above, plus officer or significant leadership position in professional organizations, or speaker at a statewide or national program.

Self Score _____ (transfer to front sheet)

Personnel Decisions to Foster Community Health   41

continued

Figure 4-3: Continued

2. Internal Leadership

A. Describe your leadership activities within Kaleida Health, but outside your direct span of control, that contribute to the growth and development of our managers and our staff. The issues listed must be demonstrated examples where you used your leadership to influence organization-wide behaviors and positions *outside* your direct area of responsibility. Do not list activities which are part of your regular job responsibilities.

Activity	Level of Participation	Demonstrate how your participation *effected* certain outcomes or evidence of your effectiveness organization-wide

B. Personal financial support of Kaleida Health fundraising efforts will be considered, if disclosed.

Kaleida Health Event Supported	$$ Range of Personal Contributions

Scale: 0 = no involvement beyond sphere of direct influence
  1 = participation as required in mandated organization-wide programs, some evidence of leadership outside direct sphere of influence.
  3 = multiple examples of significant input into organization-wide projects, educational programs; leadership provided that transcends areas of direct influence. Provides fiscal support.
  5 = awarded up to a maximum of 20 percent of eligible leaders based on senior management's assessment.

Self Score _____ (transfer to front sheet)

3. Community Service

A. Describe your ongoing efforts in serving the broader (outside Kaleida Health) community through a commitment to voluntary service. Activities must be ongoing (not single, isolated events) and applicable to your Kaleida Health job. Personal choices, such as church activities, activities associated with the employee's children, etc., are not eligible for recognition in this plan.

Activity	Level of Participation	Specifically identify the relationship of the activity to your job in Kaleida

B. Personal financial support of community fundraising events supported by Kaleida Health will be considered, if disclosed.

Community Fund Raising Event	$$ Range of Personal Contributions

Scale: 0 = no evidence of ongoing community voluntary activity.
   1 = several examples of ongoing voluntary activities with organizations whose social service missions are aligned with the Kaleida mission. Provides fiscal support.
   3 = several examples of ongoing voluntary activities, including filling a leadership role for organization(s) whose social service missions are aligned with the Kaleida mission. Provides fiscal support.
   5 = achievements as outlined in #3 above, plus community award recognition.

Self Score _____ (transfer to front sheet)

continued

FIGURE 4-3: CONTINUED

$ Range of Personal Contributions

The purpose of this chart is to allow those individuals who choose to disclose personal financial contributions made to those organizations aligned with the mission of Kaleida Health.

Using the following chart, please insert the code associated with your personal contribution under each organization.

Code	
N/A	No personal contribution made
A	$1,000 or more
B	$500–$999
C	$100–$499
D	$50–$99
E	$1–$49

encouragement ranges from providing time off to serve at state and local meetings that advance opportunities for disabled children to attending Chamber of Commerce meetings that promote economic development. Perhaps unwittingly, MHS has realized benefits from such participation, as when one MHS staff member volunteered at the regional planning council. When the community relations director sought to build a relationship with the council, the presence of the staff member helped elicit the trust of the council's executive director.

Citrus Valley Health Partners

Citrus Valley Health Partners in Covina, California, evaluates employees according to a checklist developed for their Reward and Recognition Program (see Figure 4-4). CVHP's commitment to community health is reflected in the "Community Outreach" portion of the checklist; involvement in wellness initiatives stands next to participation on committees, cost-containment suggestions, and customer service efforts.

HAVING A STABLE, LONG-TENURED EXECUTIVE TEAM

Executive turnover occurs most often in hospitals that are underutilized and have low operating margins. While some experts in management have promoted the notion that some turnover is good for organizations, in this project, the especially strong and well-balanced management teams working in sites with leading practices almost universally share unusually long tenures. Our case information suggests that it takes a few years to become highly proficient in "doing a job." From that point on, executive team members can draw on their experiences and the relationships they have built as a foundation for innovative excellence in developing practices to improve community health.

Memorial Healthcare System

Frank Sacco at Memorial Healthcare System in Hollywood, Florida, is only the third CEO to run MHS since its founding in 1947. Each of his predecessors enjoyed a long tenure in the position; the first served for 14 years and the second for 20 years. Mr. Sacco joined the MHS management team in 1974 as a department head and assumed his current role in 1987. Asked if he thought this was good for the hospital, Mr. Sacco answered, "It's good

FIGURE 4-4: CITRUS VALLEY HEALTH PARTNERS' CHECKLIST FOR
REWARD AND RECOGNITION PROGRAM

Name _____   Department _____

Soc Sec/Emp # _____   Title _____

Activity	Points	Description—Provide complete details, **attach backup** Use additional forms if needed	Total Points

EDUCATION, CERTIFICATION OR PROFESSIONAL ACTIVITIES (Attach degree, grade card, article, etc.)	1
	1
	1
	1
	1
	1
	1
		_____ Initial Certification
		_____ Degree, GED
		_____ 12 Semester Units (earned in 1997)
		_____ New Staff Orientor
		_____ Skills Day Leader
		_____ Published article
		_____ Professional organization officer
		      Organization _____
		      Office _____
		      Dates _____	

PARTICIPATION IN COMMITTEES AND TASK FORCES (See approved list of committees)	2
	
	1
		Task Forces/Committees:
		Committee _____
		   Chairperson _____
		Committee _____
		   Chairperson _____
		Committee _____
		   Chairperson _____
		
		Please list committees you were a chairperson for:
		Committee _____
		Committee _____
		Committee _____	

COMMUNITY OUTREACH	1 2	Community Health/Wellness Outreach Event (State date and individual who can verify participation) Event _____ Event _____ Event _____ Ongoing participation in Community Outreach or Partnership Program: Specify _____ Specify _____	
COST-CONTAINMENT SUGGESTION	2	Suggestion _____ _____ _____ Date Implemented _____ Suggestion _____ _____ _____ Date Implemented _____	

Activity	Points	Description—Provide complete details, **attach backup** Use additional forms if needed	Total Points
CUSTOMER SERVICE	1	Customer—Internal _____ External _____ Date _____ Unique Customer Service (Attach documentation) _____ _____ _____ _____ _____ _____	
	1	Customer—Internal _____ External _____ Date _____ Unique Customer Service (Attach documentation) _____ _____ _____ _____ _____ _____	

Maximum rewardable points = 15	Total Points	

If documentation or appropriate backup is not attached or if appropriate signatures are missing, form will be returned.

I attest that the above information is true and accurate:

_____   _____
Employee Signature   Date

_____   _____
Director   Date

_____   _____
Vice President   Date

To be completed by Human Resources:

_____   _____
Human Resources Signature   Date

Total Points Submitted _____   Total Points Denied _____   Total Points Approved _____

Comments/Reason for denial _____

_____

_____

if you've got the right people." Likewise, John Benz, strategic business and development officer, grew up in this community, knows nearly everyone in the community, and plans to retire from MHS.

Although each of the members on MHS's board have lived in the community for 20 to 25 years, their tenure has not been as long as the staff's. The board members are appointed to four-year terms with possible reappointments by Florida's governor, and only one board member remains who served when Frank Sacco became the CEO in 1987. Only two others have been on the board for as long as eight or nine years.

Mission Hospital Regional Medical Center

As do many of the leading practice sites, leadership at Mission Hospital Regional Medical Center in Mission Viejo, California, values experience and relationships. The senior management team is essentially the same team it was six years ago when Mission Hospital was owned by a group of physician-investors. The only changes in the senior management team have resulted from a retirement by the CFO and a change in CEO.

Four new senior management positions have been created. This allowed the organization to establish a better gender balance within its leadership team. Prior to the acquisition, one of the five senior management positions was held by a female. At the time of the site visit, females held five of the nine senior management positions.

Several of the senior managers noted their longevity as a team and speculated that their high standard of performance may depend in large part on their experience as a team. In addition, several senior managers expressed strong positive feelings about their association with Mission Hospital. Several noted in particular their thrill at the attention to a higher purpose, the mission of Mission Hospital that became a part of work after the Sisters of St. Joseph of Orange acquired the hospital in 1994.

Peter Bastone, the CEO, commented that six months after he arrived at Mission, others in the system asked him about his leadership team. He conducted a SWOT analysis and determined that the leadership team looked good, and after a year the system leaders had to agree. Members of the leadership team are an excellent mix of specialists. Also, the hospital has invested in human resources and benefits and are at the leading edge of benefits and pay packages—especially in Orange County.

The fact that the hospital was formerly for-profit gave it an edge that other hospitals may not have had. These managers have been challenged in a different way and have been at the hospital in both good times and bad. The COO has been particularly helpful in transitioning the organization especially vis-à-vis the physicians. The new CFO has a broad background as a hospital consultant and in the corporate sector. The continuity of leadership has made them stronger.

The long tenure of management has facilitated the development of community linkages. Kristan Schlichte, executive director of Catholic Charities in Orange County for the past 13 years, told us that her long-standing relationship with Sister Martha Ann, the hospital's vice president of sponsorship, helped her establish the Community Health Enrichment Council (CHEC) along with Bishop Driscoll, who has been the Vicar of Charities in Orange county for 28 years. This long-standing relationship among the parish, the charities, and the hospital promoted the trust that is needed for partnerships to be successful. In fact, even though the current CEO has only been formally associated with Mission Regional for three years, he has had broad experience in the Catholic health system nearby, where he worked for several years before coming to Mission.

A CEO WHO VALUES LOYALTY AND EMPOWERS STAFF

Top managers who with the CEO share a commitment to the community are the recipients of the CEO's trust and are permitted to exert much control over how to achieve the higher purposes of the organization. Such trust, in turn, produces highly motivated and skilled managers who mature with the organization and make it increasingly strong.

Citrus Valley Health Partners

Pete Makowski, CEO of Citrus Valley Health Partners, values loyalty—a feeling of mature love that can come from shared experience. This love is not just personal friendship. The ideals that cement this bond of loyalty between the CEO and key staff are their shared commitment to a higher purpose. The degree of trust engendered by this shared loyalty allows the CEO to let staff have leadership over the design of the means of achieving the higher purpose of the organization. This, in turn, engenders commitment and increasing levels of competence among the managers that are trusted. Such loyalty is akin to the bond that worshippers develop toward their faith: it binds them to their fellows and ripens into even stronger ties with time.

Indeed, the senior VP for mission integration and community care has been recruited by many individuals throughout the country, but he continues at CVHP simply because in his words, "the work is not done yet." People are given the chance to develop their job descriptions at CVHP, and this too engenders trust and loyalty. Building relationships with the community takes both commitment and time—and by rewarding loyalty, community partners are served over the long term.

EXPANDING THE ROLE OF THE HOSPITAL CEO TO INCLUDE MANAGEMENT OF PUBLIC HEALTH

During their graduate training in healthcare management, healthcare executives are taught to consider themselves as health statesmen, advocating for the health of their communities and helping to ensure that all who need healthcare are provided essential services. Their role is to support epidemiological investigations to discern threats to health in the community and to promote preventive care. Such essential public health activities are promulgated as cost-effective approaches that enable healthcare executives to realize their role. One leading practice site carried these ideas into a formal contractual relationship that allows the hospital CEO to oversee public health activities in his community.

Cambridge Health Alliance

Through a seven-year contract with the city, Cambridge Health Alliance in Cambridge, Massachussetts, provides a vast array of public health services for annual city support totaling $7.5 million. Tying public health activities with the services of an integrated delivery system has thus far served the community by attempting to ensure coordination of preventive, curative, restorative, and palliative care. The Cambridge Health Alliance enjoys a unique relationship with the community because John O'Brien, CEO for the two-hospital system, also serves as Commissioner of the Cambridge Department of Public Health.

CHAPTER FIVE

Marketing Activities that Enhance Community Health

INPUT—LISTENING TO the voice the community—and output—reporting back—are elements of contemporary marketing found to be practiced in old and new ways at leading hospitals. Practices that effect this strategy include surveys and interviews to help hospitals learn about health assets and issues in the community. Reporting out can remind employers and taxpayers that hospitals are there to promote health and improve residents' quality of life. We learned that leading hospitals sometimes take a very quiet, self-effacing role in partnering with others. They also celebrate the achievements of community health activists.

COLLECTING COMMUNITY HEALTH INFORMATION

Community health assessments are necessary to understand the community's health status and to learn about the larger environment within which the organization operates.

Data such as the demographic and socioeconomic characteristics as well as health status and risks to health can help inform other data. To be most useful, this information should be collected over time—at least every five years—so that trends can be observed. Hospitals and health systems that do not use community health data as part of their direction-setting process are behind the curve in terms of market awareness and discovering synergies between organizational strategies and other initiatives in the area. Hospitals need not necessarily collect their own data; they can use information gathered by other agencies or work collaboratively. In fact, in many communities, duplicative assessments are still the norm. Leading practice sites have developed a tradition of conducting such assessments collaboratively—with public health agencies, other hospitals, community agencies such as the United Way or Catholic Charities, or a consortium of such agencies.

LINKING STRATEGY WITH COMMUNITY HEALTH THROUGH DATA

Mission Hospital Regional Medical Center

In 1995, Mission Hospital Regional Medical Center in Mission Viejo, California, initiated a yearlong community health assessment. As a result of California SB 697 community benefit legislation, an assessment was required by the summer of 1996; however, Mission had started its assessment prior to passage of SB 697.

This 1995 assessment involved two committees. One was a blue ribbon panel of mayors, agency heads, and business leaders. This group served mainly to grease wheels, to lend credibility, and to ensure that the assessment avoided political challenges. The other committee was a working committee, including staff from local colleges, utility companies, civic organizations, social services organizations, and others. The goal in composing this second group was to involve anyone who was already working with the community, to include as much local intelligence as possible from the very outset.

The 1995 assessment included a telephone survey of 400 residents of Mission Viejo and Laguna Niguel. These two cities comprised 37 percent of the hospital's patient service area. The survey results were used to determine an appropriate design for focus groups with citizens about the causes of the problems and issues identified by the survey. The focus groups were followed by key informant interviews that were intended mainly to flesh out the team's understanding of the issues and their causes.

As a result of the 1995 surveys, Mission Hospital's Community Benefit Committee established its priorities in care for the poor. These priorities led to investments in senior transportation, pediatric dental care at the Camino Clinic, and the Family Resource Center.

A new assessment was launched by the county in 1998. Forty-two hospitals, including Mission Hospital, contributed $2,500 each to underwrite the county health department's efforts in this assessment. This assessment used three different instruments, all by telephone interview. These instruments assessed (1) behavioral health, (2) physical health, and (3) quality of life and personal behavior. The data collection phase was completed in the summer of 1998.

Unfortunately, the county's contract with California State University at Fullerton did not anticipate the need for data analysis and reporting. Hence,

Mission Hospital is now determining how it can help the county conduct analyses and produce local reports. Local reports will focus on the three poorest cities in Mission Hospital's service area: Dana Point, San Clemente, and San Juan Capistrano. So far, St. Joseph's health system, with which Mission Hospital is affiliated, is loaning a statistician to the county so that small-area analyses can be completed and reports generated for the participating hospitals.

Meanwhile, three organizations partnered to win a grant from Orange County for the purposes of canvassing low-income communities. Catholic Charities, The Mission of San Juan Capistrano, and Mission Hospital partnered to form the Community Health Enrichment Council (CHEC). CHEC designed and oversaw a door-to-door quality of life assessment in the poorest neighborhoods of their service area. California State University at Fullerton received a contract to hire and train local residents from these neighborhoods to conduct the surveys.

As a result of this survey on quality of life, CHEC is designing materials on parenting skills in Spanish and investigating how to deliver these materials to the poorest neighborhoods. Such materials are already being delivered in English to other parts of the service area. CHEC will also use the data to design other programs for the poorest neighbors.

EMBEDDING VALUES ABOUT COMMUNITY HEALTH IN ONGOING STRATEGY

Memorial Healthcare System

Memorial Healthcare System in Hollywood, Florida, cooperates with other organizations, notably the Coordinating Council of Broward County, to conduct periodic telephone interviews designed to learn what the sampled 2,000 county residents feel about the state of families and communities, safety, education, the local economy, environment, government, and healthcare. The survey report provides trend information for the county and comparative information for the state of Florida. In addition, goals are projected for the years 2000 and 2010.

Other data are collected by census tract. These data enable the hospital to track community needs and are used in conjunction with focus groups of residents to lend reality to the information.

Once data are collected, the Coordinating Council of Broward compiles "The Broward Benchmarks," a publication that reports the following statistics (among many others):

- The percentage of low birth weight babies for whites, non-whites, and collectively

- The percentage of at-risk mothers receiving prenatal screening
- The percentage of at-risk newborns receiving infant screening
- The percentage of uninsured people, by age
- The race of nonelderly adults (18–64 yrs) who are uninsured (white, non-white, and from a Spanish-speaking country)
- The level of satisfaction of those receiving healthcare
- The preventable cancer death rate (county and state)
- The percentage of early-stage breast cancer diagnoses (county and state)
- The percentage of early-stage prostate cancer diagnoses (county and state)
- The percentage of adults who had a medical check-up in the previous year
- The percentage of women over age 50 who had mammograms in the past year and both mammograms and clinical breast exams in the previous two years
- The percentage of people, by age, who had a dental checkup within the previous year
- The percentage of adults who practice safe sex.

MHS leaders advise that strategic plans serve a community health perspective better when they are less focused on a set of specific community health status measures. They prefer instead to use a broad array of health and quality of life information. Memorial's use of community quality of life data for direction setting and performance monitoring started through United Way's Compass methodology. MHS then contracted with David Smith, of Smith Abt, to conduct a Community Health Needs Analysis. This effort started with South Broward County but was expanded to include both South and North Broward Counties.

CONNECTING TO THE COMMUNITY THROUGH INTERVIEWS

Connecting to the community through interviews involves hospital representatives becoming acquainted with both the key health problems in the community and the local leaders who could help solve them. Starting with groups that the hospital representatives know, each is asked to identify not only the community's problems they perceive but also experts who know a good deal about them. This "reputational approach" allows the hospital to connect to more and more individuals and groups.

Memorial Healthcare System

Every community action organization experiments with ways to identify and engage citizens or neighborhood leaders who might otherwise be unknown to a hospital or health system. Memorial Healthcare System in Hollywood, Florida, has used a method that involved inviting groups of known community leaders from specific areas to "two for $13" lunches at a local restaurant. These groups are asked to answer two questions: (1) What are the top three problems in our community?, and (2) Who in our community knows more about this than I do? The second of these questions identifies people to be invited to lunch.

With each progressive cycle of identifying problems and leaders, three outcomes are achieved: (1) confirmation of the top community issues that need resolution, (2) identification of new leaders who could help solve the problems, and (3) acquainting local opinion leaders with MHS's efforts to understand issues from their perspective. Hence, the circle of participation has grown, as has local support for MHS's effort. As the cycle continues, the top problems become clearer, setting the stage for efforts to engage local partners in ways to address those problems.

Using this approach, John Benz, senior VP for mission integration and community care, determined that in MHS's primary services area (South Broward County), getting jobs was a key issue. He then used total quality management techniques to determine what prevented people from obtaining and keeping jobs. Using a fishbone diagram, Mr. Benz and his group of community advisers found that the lack of east-west public transportation presented a major barrier for many job seekers. Therefore transportation became the key agenda item for countywide resolution.

Citrus Valley Health Partners

At the outset of his new responsibilities as senior VP of mission integration and community care at Citrus Valley Health Partners in Covina, California, Tom McGuiness began an ongoing practice of conducting one-on-one interviews with colleagues, partners, prospective partners, and others. He has conducted over 900 of these interviews. One of Mr. McGuiness' main questions is: "Who are the people in the community that can make your dream for a healthier community come true?"

Every participating partner had one of these interviews early in its relationship with CVHP. Moreover, informants in his community hold that these ongoing interactions produce numerous opportunities for synergies. Mr. McGuiness's role became one of messenger, which entailed mixing and matching information from various sources, sorting it into usable bundles, and feeding it back to various partners and potential partners through other interviews or meetings.

The 900 interviews conducted by Tom McGuiness served as the launching point through which CVHP could listen to the community's wishes. The interviews were followed with lunches, and meetings were facilitated by content specialists.

Through its outreach efforts, CVHP actively seeks ways to bridge to others to better provide services in ways that plug gaps and, more importantly, deepen and broaden the community's capacities to serve one another. In part, this role includes putting up seed money. However, Mr. McGuiness and CEO Peter Makowski both stress that CVHP will only provide start-up funds. Ultimately, projects that are supported have to be self-sustaining. Other principles CVHP emphasizes at these meetings include teaching partners to use a common language. CVHP attempts to be a low-cost vendor of choice for safety net providers by using the down time of their services and equipment, such as lab, mammography, and radiology, and thus increase access to care for the poor and uninsured. Through such efforts, CVHP attempts to prove its trustworthiness. Typically multiple staff and board members are able to engage directly in the partners' work or joint activities. However, community relationships must not be undertaken for public relations or marketing purposes. Instead, these relationships are the essence of how the health system lives with and serves its community.

LESSONS FROM THE DEMONSTRATION SITES

Kaleida Health

Kaleida Health in Buffalo, New York, now provides a report about community health objectives to its board through its planning committee. Such data are used in board meetings. Efforts are now underway to prepare a brief overview of the major Kaleida activities so that the board gets a sense of the many and varied partnerships underway.

ISSUING REPORT CARDS

Report cards on community health performance can take various forms: a brochure, a newspaper insert, or a poster that is widely distributed to the community. Report cards describe a number of recent health measures about the community. Often the report card presents data from prior years, goals or targets for the present and future years, and/or national data for comparative purposes.

Cambridge Health Alliance

A report card issued by Cambridge Health Alliance in Cambridge, Massachussetts, showing community health statistics for the communities of Cambridge and Somerville and comparing the two communities to Massachusetts and *Healthy People 2000* benchmarks, is published and widely disseminated every year. The report card, in an approach borrowed from Marion County, Indiana, gives information on 16 different indicators in six different areas:

1. Access to health and prevention services
2. Encouraging healthier behaviors
3. Preventing violence
4. Reducing injury
5. Reducing substance abuse
6. Preventing AIDS and other STDs

Indicators, based largely on data available from primary and secondary sources, include cigarette smoking in the past 30 days by children, grades 9 through 12; immunization rates by age 2; deaths due to cancer per 100,000; and the number of persons with AIDS in the community.

Prior to the merger with Cambridge Hospital that founded the Alliance, Somerville Hospital had done a comprehensive evaluation of community health as part of the Somerville Community Health Agenda process in the early 1990s. Somerville has repeated its assessments every two years since then. Cambridge started conducting similar assessments from 1994 to 1997. However, these data were not used for a community report card, a format designed for easy access and use by the general public, until 1998. More recent assessments include thorough reports on the plans for action that result from the community health assessments and accompanying review of results by the various partners in the community.

Camcare, Inc.

Camcare, Inc.'s employees in Charleston, West Virginia, have learned that the organization, working through its individual staff members, is committed to delivering increased value through improvements in quality, service, and cost. Through its annual Report Card, Camcare publicly accounts for its progress in improving its structures, processes, and outcomes relative to community health.

The Report Card is a product derived from a much more comprehensive and detailed reporting mechanism, the Camcare System Performance

Indicators. These measures, in turn, are indicators that track progress toward accomplishment of the four enduring goals in the Camcare Strategic Plan: 1) to be an integrator of care; 2) to be a seamless system; 3) to *measurably* improve quality; and 4) to improve community health status. Annually, Report Cards are mailed to purchasers of Camcare services such as members of the Chamber of Commerce, insurance companies, public agencies, and other healthcare systems. In 1999, Camcare prepared an advertisement-style Report Card to be placed in local newspapers so community residents could have access to this information.

The enduring goals of Camcare's strategic plan align with the incentives present in a prudent purchaser market. Annual incentive payments to executives and managers of Camcare also align, as they are partially contingent on achieving both corporate and individual objectives related to the enduring goals. By "drilling down" expectations and incentives to the department manager level, Camcare's leadership has created virtually universal understanding among its staff of the objectives, measures, and personal contributions required to realize the mission of Camcare. Since 1996, all redesign efforts have focused on improving quality, service, or cost, and thereby enhancing value. At the department level, specific, measurable objectives are developed. Staff of Camcare learn of achievement through the quarterly and annual System Performance Indicator reports. The community learns of achievement through the Camcare Health System Report Cards that are published. Both documents deal with patient satisfaction, for example, but the system performance indicators are much more detailed. Other highly readable information concerns comparisons of average charges for a variety of DRGs.

Crozer-Keystone Health System

Crozer-Keystone Health System in Media, Pennsylvania, distributes attractive brochures displaying colorful, easy-to-read graphics that report community health statistics. Figure 5-1 is just one example of the reporting that is published on that community's health.

LESSONS LEARNED FROM THE DEMONSTRATION SITES

Evergreen Community Health Care

Evergreen Community Health Care developed a 15-page report and a one-page summary detailing the results of ECHC's many collaborative community initiatives. The latter was extremely well received by board members. Also, the report in the hospital's newsletter focused on mortality and morbidity statistics. Some thought this should be expanded to include other

Reducing Risk for Cancer
Preventive Screenings

	'92	'94	'96	National Goal*	
Breast Exam Females 18+	70%	72%	75%	60%	☺
Prostate Exam Males 50+	NA	67%	70%	40%	☺
Colorectal Exam Adults	NA	41%	50%	50%	☺
Mammogram Females 50+	NA	71%	74%	60%	☺
PAP Smear Females 18+	NA	81%	82%	85%	☹

Healthy People 2000: National Health Promotion Objectives

measures in the future, especially measures of preventive programs like "Teens Being Valued," as well as outcomes information.

MULTI-BRANDING—PROMOTING COMMUNITY HEALTH WITH AND THROUGH PARTNERS

Multi-branding happens when a hospital or system invests money, expertise, or other resources into a community health program, but does not advertise its involvement. Community health ideas and programs that the hospital or system promotes are carried out under the name of both the hospital and its partner, under the brand name of other community organizations exclusively, or under the name of a community health concept or program. This approach enables the hospital to work in the background, but it also focuses more attention on the community health program itself. Hospitals therefore maintain the trust of their partners by avoiding using community health programs to increase utilization of their service.

Memorial Hospital and Health System

Memorial Hospital and Health System's partners explain that although they received support from Memorial, their projects were consistently identified as their own. Memorial was rarely identified as a partner. Even though Memorial's marketing department spends as much as 25 percent of their time on community health projects, the Memorial logo is nowhere to be found. Yet most community leaders know that Memorial is partnering with many of these agencies. On some projects, the B.A.B.E. program for example, Memorial works with its competitors.

Beds and Britches Etc. (B.A.B.E.) is an incentive program for perinatal care in which pregnant women and new mothers receive vouchers from participating physicians and social services agencies throughout St. Joseph County. B.A.B.E. stores, located throughout St. Joseph County in non-Memorial clinical and agency settings, offer new and used clothing for babies and young children and equipment including cribs, car seats, and toys. Merchandise is obtained through coupons distributed by local collaborating agencies. The program has been adopted by many other communities.

Memorial Hospital and Health System also partners with the Center for the Homeless, which provides a step-by-step process to move individuals and families from emergency shelter to homeownership (see Figure 5-2). Memorial underwrites the health programs of the South Bend homeless shelter. Not only do they provide medical care, they also negotiate arrangements that help teach valuable skills to the homeless residents. For example, Memoral partnered with ServiceMaster to train the homeless residents on how to provide lawn care services. Now, all lawn care services for the hospital are supplied by the workers of the homeless shelter. Ultimately, the goal is to teach residents life-sustaining skills so that they can hold down good jobs and own their own home.

Camcare, Inc.

Camcare, Inc. in Charleston, West Virginia, has acted as an incubator for a community health agenda, which has led to a number of ways of "selling" the idea of community health. The Kanawha Coalition for Community Health Improvement is one of several means by which Camcare can participate in community health–oriented work without branding the activity as the system's. Camcare was a major force behind the launch of the Coalition, paying two-thirds of the coordinator's salary and operating expenses through the CAMC Foundation. However, in the interest of enjoying a neutral and equitable framework for community health efforts, Camcare has deliberately avoided promoting its own corporate identity in these efforts.

The Coalition, on the other hand, is recognized by opinion leaders in the community as a neutral ground for joint leadership on community

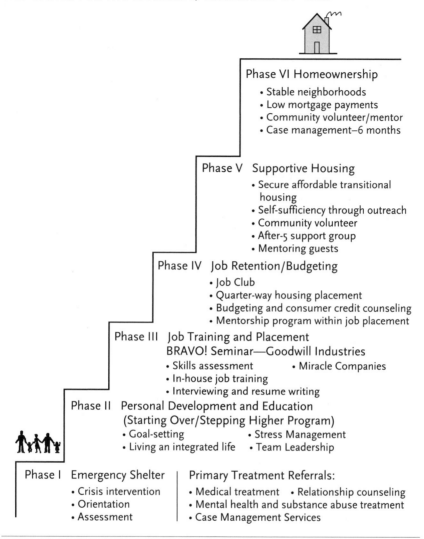

Phase VI Homeownership
- Stable neighborhoods
- Low mortgage payments
- Community volunteer/mentor
- Case management–6 months

Phase V Supportive Housing
- Secure affordable transitional housing
- Self-sufficiency through outreach
- Community volunteer
- After-5 support group
- Mentoring guests

Phase IV Job Retention/Budgeting
- Job Club
- Quarter-way housing placement
- Budgeting and consumer credit counseling
- Mentorship program within job placement

**Phase III Job Training and Placement
BRAVO! Seminar—Goodwill Industries**
- Skills assessment
- In-house job training
- Interviewing and resume writing
- Miracle Companies

**Phase II Personal Development and Education
(Starting Over/Stepping Higher Program)**
- Goal-setting
- Living an integrated life
- Stress Management
- Team Leadership

Phase I Emergency Shelter
- Crisis intervention
- Orientation
- Assessment

Primary Treatment Referrals:
- Medical treatment
- Relationship counseling
- Mental health and substance abuse treatment
- Case Management Services

and community health issues. The Coalition allows all partners to participate on the basis of an equal voice and stake. Priorities established by the
community for the Coalition include tobacco use, heart disease, and lack
of physical activity. Outside of the Coalition, community health efforts for
the system have focused on extending the health improvement process to
other areas such as Fayette County, working to measure community health
processes and outcomes with the Partners in Health Network, focusing

Marketing Activities that Enhance Community Health   61

on the African-American population through the church community, and other local neighborhood efforts.

Camcare has also been an important partner in the background for Health Right, a free clinic. Camcare has contributed financial support, pharmacy services, physician services, and volunteers. Camcare also provided space to Health Right at its inception, as well as construction support during remodeling of Health Right's facility. Health Right receives the bulk of its financial support from private sources, including the other two hospitals in the area. Health Right has been successfully duplicated in five other communities throughout the state.

Citrus Valley Health Partners

Citrus Valley Health Partners has championed the Family Resource Center Collaborative in its community. With the support of the East San Gabriel Valley Community Health Council and foundations, civic groups, local institutions and businesses, municipalities, and private individuals, the Collaborative has established Family Resource Centers, described as community hubs and integration points to deliver services to residents. Figure 5-3 highlights the services the centers provide and lists the major initiatives of the Collaborative in 1998 and 1999.

CONNECTING TO CONSUMERS THROUGH INFORMATION SYSTEMS

Using techniques ranging from published directories to e-mail, healthcare systems are attempting to provide various segments of the community with general health information as well as information about available health providers. Information systems also allow healthcare organizations to inform specific segments of the community about available resources such as childhood immunizations, senior health screenings, and support group availability.

Crozer-Keystone Health System

Crozer-Keystone Health System in Media, Pennsylvania, has aggressively pursued the use of new information technology to gather information from and get information to special groups of citizens. These efforts create the expectation of a community health focus among staff and the public. The first of these efforts was the creation of a directory of all the health and

Types of FRC Services

- Affordable/free primary medical, dental, pharmacy care
- Affordable/free individual and family counseling
- Food, clothing, housing, and transportation assistance
- Welfare-to-work and related employment skills training
- Substance abuse referral services
- Community outreach services
- Assistance applying for economic aid and social services
- Children's after-school tutoring and recreation programs
- Public health services and immunizations
- Adult education and English as a Second Language (ESL)
- Assistance applying for U.S. citizenship and voter registration
- Mentoring and academic assistance
- Parenting skills classes
- Wellness, illness prevention, and nutrition programs
- Domestic violence intervention and prevention

Major Initiatives

- Continued development and implementation of an integrated strategic plan and integrated decision making
- Development of community-wide health, human services, and civic services outreach networks
- Establishment of a regional information system enabling FRCs to share appropriate client, program, clinical, educational, needs, and service capacity information
- Replication of successful core programs and services at all FRCs while elimination of service duplication
- Expansion of the network of partnerships with providers, communities, institutions, and volunteers to ensure a seamless continuum of care and services in each community
- Assistance of FRCs in developing economic sustainability plans to reduce disproportionate reliance on grant and government funding
- Development of additional partnerships and programs supporting legislative initiatives such as Healthy Families, GAIN and Welfare Reform
- Assistance of other communities desiring support in establishing Family Resource Centers

human services in the area. These *Green Pages* also offer a lot of basic information about health and healthcare topics like patients' rights, how often to have cholesterol levels checked and how to lower them, as well as stress management techniques. Under "dermatology," for example, the *Green Pages* includes a general definition of the specialty, a phone number for more information, and a listing of community resources, including a description and contact information for the Scleroderma Federation of the Delaware Valley. Other entries might include a listing of Crozer-Keystone programs and phone numbers.

The child health database represents one of the returns Crozer-Keystone receives for its investment in information systems. About 4,000 births are recorded per year. Crozer-Keystone communicates advisories every two months, informing consumers about immunizations that should be scheduled. As of the time of our visit, about 25,000 infants had been logged into this registry.

Crozer-Keystone has obtained a $224,000 grant from the Department of Commerce to provide seniors access to technology. Seniors are being given access to computers and the training to use them. Part of the hardware solution is the acquisition of off-the-shelf equipment like computers and WebTV consoles. The entry point into this senior information system is Crozer-Keystone's web page. The Crozer-Keystone web page (www.crozer.org) includes the *Green Pages* and has a number of hyperlinks to other resources such as the Social Security Administration. It also allows seniors to communicate with their own caregivers. Perhaps most engaging for many seniors is that this system gives them e-mail access to their friends and children, bolstering seniors' social support networks. Crozer-Keystone also operates a Call Center, which provides another means of accessing the information found in the *Green Pages*.

As part of this investment in consumer information systems, Crozer-Keystone has helped acquire computers for use by children participating in the programs of the Chester Education Foundation. Crozer-Keystone is also one of a number of partners building a Smart Building, which is being prepared to house product and business innovations by high-tech firms, health systems, and universities.

In the future, Crozer-Keystone expects to use push technology to target specific audiences and to make these information resources more interactive.

Camcare, Inc.

Camcare, Inc. conducts quarterly reporting on a wide array of performance indicators, including many related to community health. The Camcare

System Performance Indicators Report is organized around the four enduring goals of the system. These four goals are repeated below, with illustrative performance measures given for each:

1. To position the Camcare system as the region's cost-effective integrator of quality care capable of simplicity, stability, and competence to the purchasers of healthcare.
   a) CAMC Return on Assets
   b) Carelink Market Share
   c) Carelink Member Satisfaction
   d) Primary Care Physicians to Population
2. To operate Camcare as a seamless system.
   a) CAMC Regional Charge Comparison
   b) CAMC Average Length of Stay
   c) CAMC Medicare/Medicaid Unreimbursed Services
   d) CAMC ER Utilization
3. To enhance the efficiency and effectiveness of our services as demonstrated through measurable quality improvements.
   a) Camcare Employee Opinion Survey
   b) CAMC Community Opinion Survey Results
   c) Carelink Customer Service
   d) CAMC Unscheduled Readmission Rate
   e) CAMC Appropriateness of Care/Breast Biopsies
4. To improve the health status of the communities we serve.
   a) Health Risk Appraisals
   b) Community Health Assessment
   c) Carelink Population-Based Indicators
   d) CAMC Community Health Education/Screening

About 50 indicators are regularly tracked. The indicators are reported at different intervals, some quarterly (such as patient satisfaction), some semiannually, and some annually. This staggered tracking and reporting of indicators makes for a more manageable process; it also enhances the system's ability to make use of the data in educational efforts with board members, physician leaders, and the community overall.

Camcare uses Lyons Software's community benefit reporting software, developed by the VHA and the Catholic Health Association. Camcare also conducts a Community Leadership Profile, which logs the organization, type of work, number of hours, and estimated economic value of voluntary labor given by Camcare employees to community organizations. Managers are encouraged to support their employees in volunteering to work with community organizations.

HOLDING RECOGNITION EVENTS TO HONOR COMMUNITY HEALTH ACTIVISTS

Recognition events publicly honor individuals who act as catalysts for the hospital or system to improve internal management and care systems as well as outreach and partnership efforts so the hospital or system can better promote community health. These events can be conducted as "summits," employee recognition programs, or any number of other programs.

Mission Hospital Regional Medical Center

Sister Martha Ann, as vice president of sponsorship at Mission Hospital, promotes the mission, vision, and values of the organization. For example, she serves as the hospital's representative on several system-level committees: on the Healthy Communities Roundtable, the Sponsorship Executive Committee, and other ad hoc committees.

The Healthy Communities Roundtable meets semiannually to discuss best practices among the system entities and held a Healthy Community Summit in March 1999. This Summit asked each hospital to prepare a video of its accomplishments in improving one quality of life indicator—for example, safety, education, healthcare, clean water, or employment—for the members of their communities. Each hospital sent 20 representatives to the Summit, and hospitals were publicly recognized for their improvement efforts.

Another committee that Sister Martha Ann sits on at the system level is the Sponsorship Executive Committee. This committee sponsors a recognition program called Values in Action, which recognizes those who embody the core values of the Sisters of St. Joseph's of Orange system. The committee also considers policies and procedures that help to advance the mission and values by promoting the orientation program (see chapter 3). The goal of the system is to encourage all their hospitals in the various communities to embrace the concept of healthy communities.

CHAPTER SIX

Creating Structures that Institutionalize Attention to Community Health

L EADING HOSPITALS SHOWED us that instead of relying on ap-pointed individuals to carry out community missions, they could in-stitutionalize their commitment to community health by creating a special organizational unit. Units serve to gather and analyze data, recruit fund-raisers, teach future leaders, educate the board and the community, and generate ideas to effect the hospital's community health programs. Spe-cialized units of the hospital with cogent statements of function enable them to help keep the hospital's feet to the fire and promote its community health vision.

CREATING A HEALTH INFORMATION UNIT THAT SUPPORTS COMMUNITY HEALTH

Some hospitals and health systems have established a specialized depart-ment that aggregates secondary (previously collected) data and sometimes primary data to describe community health and track performance. Health units ideally incorporate public health measures, private healthcare mea-sures, and more general quality of life information in their reports. The capacity to organize such data and see the interplay between public health issues, healthcare services, and quality of life can serve a large partnership, as well as the individual organizations participating in the partnership.

Cambridge Health Alliance

The Cambridge Health Alliance in Cambridge, Massachussetts, has created a health information unit that is part of the public health department. Using largely public sources of data, the unit collects information about the health status of the communities of Somerville and Cambridge. The unit also assists Somerville in the collection, organization, and analysis of community health data for that city. The unit offers technical skills and report development and production for both cities. The unusual relationship between the public authority that oversees healthcare delivery and the Cambridge Public Health Department (John O'Brien is CEO of the Cambridge Health Alliance and the commissioner of public health for Cambridge) makes this unit for improving the community-wide healthcare delivery system especially useful. The unit reflects a very high degree of integration between medicine and public health.

DEVELOPING AN INSTITUTE FOR COMMUNITY HEALTH

Based on the concept of the think tank in a retreat-like setting, an Institute for Community Health typically has a mission to engage community leaders in a dialog to develop a vision and enhance leadership capacities to effect change.

Citrus Valley Health Partners

The Institute for Community Leadership at Citrus Valley Health Partners in Covina, California was formally launched a week prior to our site visit. The Institute's mission is "to enhance leadership capacity by educating and strengthening community leaders toward the transformation of their communities." CVHP, along with three universities and the Department of Health Services, provided start-up funds for the Institute, which consists of four initiatives:

1. Leadership conferences where nationally recognized speakers are brought in to speak to the leaders in the public and private sectors,
2. A two-year academy that offers eight courses as follow-ups to the leadership conference,
3. An oral archives program that captures the stories of community leaders, and
4. A sabbatical residential program for community leaders (six to eight weeks to think, rest, reflect, study, and write).

The Institute is seen as a "Santa Fe Institute" for the community. Instead of having people listen to lectures, dialog is sought to develop a vision and leadership skills.

The idea of the Institute arose from the one-on-one interviews that Tom McGuiness, senior VP for mission integration and community care, conducted with members of his community, during which it became evident that individuals had great passion and capacities and wanted training. John Suggs, the Institute's regional consultant, had experience helping leaders envision the future in post-apartheid South Africa. The Institute presents an opportunity for him to facilitate leaders' future thinking in Southern California.

CVHP, the Los Angeles County Health Department, and several universities, including the UCLA School of Public Health, Immaculate Heart College Center, and the University of La Verne, are collaborating in the Institute. Both UCLA and the county bought into the project based on a personal trust that was built over time with Mr. McGuiness. CVHP had done much of the groundwork in identifying the needs for the Institute.

The partners first worked on the Institute's foundational principles and emerged with 16 principles that are based on the fundamental belief that all resources and systems should serve to enhance and strengthen healthier communities. For example, the principle on women is that "the spirit and power of women's voices are equally valued." Interestingly, one of the potential partners objected to this principle but Mr. Suggs maintained that it was fundamental to the partners' agreement and insisted it remain a tenet. When told that the principle on women was questioned, another partner stated that if it had been removed or even weakened, that partner would have withdrawn. Thus, the Institute walks a tightrope trying to advance community leadership capacities while maintaining internal integrity.

Underlying the Institute's approach is the concept of respecting individuals' experiences. The concept is based in part on Miles Horton's views as embodied in the Highlander Community—a training ground established in the 1950s and a program that civil rights leaders Rosa Parks and Martin Luther King, Jr. attended.

CVHP put up the first money for the Institute—and for a long time theirs was the only money for the project. These funds provided the Institute organizers with organizational and financial credibility, and ultimately helped to bring the other partners along. Of those currently going through the academy, 16 slots are filled by the county and 6 slots are filled by CVHP.

In addition to the initial planners, who are the core instructors of the academy, the outside instructors include local experts who receive a small stipend for their contribution. The Institute holds all of its Conference and academy sessions in community settings—in schools, hospitals, and similar buildings, not in hotels. More information about the Institute can be found at its website, www.ph.ucla.edu.icl.

ESTABLISHING A COMMITTEE OF THE BOARD TO DISCUSS QUALITY AND COMMUNITY HEALTH

All hospital boards have committees with quality oversight responsibilities. Since quality usually focuses on clinical outputs, enlarging the focus to include population and community health is a reasonable next step for organizations with well-functioning quality oversight committees. Such a board committee, sometimes chaired by a physician, becomes able to consider quality of care issues from a system and community perspective. The reports this committee generates to the full board can form the basis of "report cards" provided to the community. Although the reports often span one calendar year, another leading practice is to provide rolling three-year measurements that better reflect the long lead times needed to observe community health outcomes.

Crozer-Keystone Health System

Reflecting its focus on the new banner of a community health system, in 1996 Crozer-Keystone in Media, Pennsylvania, commissioned a committee of the board to reconsider the organization's approaches to quality. The result was a board committee that in addition to patient care quality and medical staff credentialing reviews the organization's performance on quality of care issues from a system- and health-management perspective. The co-chairs, Robert Welsh and Joseph Stock, M.D., agreed to lead this committee with the stipulation that it not be relegated to playing second fiddle to the finance committee's reports at the board meetings. The Crozer-Keystone board is now striving to adjust its agenda and reporting practices so that the quality of care committee gets equal time with the finance committee.

Many indices tracked by this board committee measure quality from a community health perspective and are reported quarterly to the system board. The "First Annual Report on Quality, Fiscal Year 1998" included a number of measures that are benchmarked against *Healthy People 2000* objectives. The report notes that 72 percent of the people over 65 years old in their managed care population received influenza immunizations, which exceeds the *Healthy People 2000* goal of 60 percent for this age cohort. Crozer-Keystone also exceeded *Healthy People 2000* goals in blood pressure and cholesterol screenings, regular exercise by adults, breast exams, prostate exams, colorectal exams, mammograms, routine medical and dental exams for children, seat belt use, and bicycle helmet use. Crozer-Keystone continues trying to improve community health performance in terms of the percentage of females who get pap smears and the percentage of adults who smoke.

The board is now considering the use of rolling three-year measurements instead of just tracking a single year's performance. Some of the population and community health indicators Crozer-Keystone is tracking are not very sensitive to change within one year. In addition, the heavy demands on communication with the community for some of the initiatives require months just to get started, and the eventual rewards of such efforts simply cannot be observed within one year.

The system produces and publishes reports on quality intended for consumers. These reports are very consumer friendly. Produced on card stock in a 3-by-9-inch 12-page brochure, they are brief and attractive with plenty of white space. The reports use icons of smiling faces to show where goals have been met and frowning faces where they have not (see Figure 5-1). An even briefer communication of performance was produced and disseminated as *Focus on Community Health* in the spring of 1998.

For example, a report tracks the death rate in Delaware County and the United States from 1991 through 1995 as well as leading causes of death and the improvement over time of blood pressure and cholesterol screenings. One useful section discusses improving maternal and child health and compares, for example, the national goal of 50 percent of children using bicycle helmets to the 65 percent actually attained in Delaware County.

LESSONS LEARNED FROM THE DEMONSTRATION SITES

St. Mary Medical Center

St. Mary Medical Center in Hobart, Indiana, was able to integrate its own board into the healthy community process by having the board's quality committee report at each meeting on issues relating to community health. In addition, the CEO added the annual goals for community initiatives to the summary report provided to each board member at its bimonthly meeting. A final planned element is for the head of the board's quality committee to be appointed to the Community Health Council, a group of community leaders whose role is to decide on the priorities to pursue to make Hobart a healthier community.

INCLUDING STAFF ON BOARD COMMITTEES

Board committees may be chaired by board members but composed almost entirely of senior managers and physicians. Such staff participation greatly increases the board's access to accurate and thorough information and produces a more collaborative climate between the board and the senior managers.

Memorial Healthcare System

The Memorial Healthcare System board, as a public institution in Hollywood, Florida, operates under strong sunshine provisions; that is, meetings must be open to the public. In addition, the board by-laws call for only seven members. Moreover, with its commitment to community health and quality of life, MHS pursues a broad agenda. To meet the objectives related to these circumstances, the MHS leadership has adopted a staff-intensive board committee model.

MHS has 14 board committees. Each committee is chaired by a board member. At any point in time, most board members chair two committees. The remainder of each committee, however, is made up of senior management, including the CEO, and the hospital's physician leadership.

This tight bond between senior management and individual board members apparently increases the board's access to accurate and thorough information, and enables them to be more familiar with management's efforts to implement the board's strategic directions. Moreover, board members serve as content experts to the whole board and sometimes as representatives of the hospital to other community agencies.

For example, Mary Washington is the chair of the board's community relations committee. In her regular daytime work as the director of the Hallendale Center for Human Services, which provides after-school programs for children, 4-H clubs, nutrition programs, and other services, Ms. Washington is in contact with many individuals in need. Most recently, she has become aware that while the primary care clinics located in the health department are now well-staffed and open to the public for extended hours and on the weekends, the clinic itself is inaccessible by public transportation. She has become involved as one of the MHS representatives with the Coalition for a Healthy South Broward—a group of civic-minded individuals representing various community groups. At the meeting we attended, Ms. Washington praised the transportation department officials who were attempting to provide greater public transportation access to these clinics.

Overall, fixing individual board member accountability has fostered active, involved governance with dedicated and knowledgeable staff to promote MHS's community-oriented goals. The minutes of a meeting of the community relations committee displayed in Figure 6-1 demonstrate the activities and the effectiveness of this committee.

Group: COMMUNITY RELATIONS COMMITTEE   *Date:* November 17, 1998
Chairman: Mary Washington   *Time:* 4 p.m.
Location: Executive Conference Room

Ms. Washington opened the meeting and welcomed all attendees.

A. Community Benefits

Memorial's Community Benefits Department, along with Modello Park residents and other community groups, joined together to demolish two crack homes and help clean up (beautify) the Modello Park area. The Senior Program members have been sewing clothes and refurbishing toys to give to needy families for the holidays. The Intergeneration Program is working to rebuild trust and bridge the generation gap between teens and seniors in Modello Park.

B. Community Relations

More than 1,000 South Broward children received free immunizations, hearing and vision screenings, and school physicals through our Back-to-School Readiness Program. A Back-to-School clothing drive provided more than 550 children with new clothes and shoes. In recognition of Breast Cancer Awareness month (October), seven Purple Teas were conducted where several hundred women received instruction on cancer prevention and breast self-examination. Initiated a program offering flu shots at eight locations throughout South Broward. Secured $31,000 in grants for community outreach programs.

C. Public Relations

Received regional and national media coverage on a rare bone transplant surgery that was performed for the first time in the United States by Dr. Michael Jofe at the Joe DiMaggio Children's Hospital. Additionally, achieved extensive media coverage for the Memorial Regional Heart Institute's four surgeons as well as on pediatric cardiac surgery and pediatric interventional cardiac catheterization programs.

D. Marketing

Implemented a strong campaign announcing Memorial Hospital Pembroke's Accreditation with Commendation and its ranking in the top four percent of hospitals nationwide. Implemented award campaigns recognizing Joe DiMaggio Children's Hospital's being voted Best Children's Hospital and Memorial Hospital West's awards for Most Family Friendly Employer, Best Hospital/ Maternity, Best Gym in South Florida, and Best Women's Center. Also developed a high-tech campaign for Memorial Regional Heart Institute and its nationally renowned heart surgeons.

E. Coalition for a Healthy South Broward

This is a powerful and diverse group of people in the community who have come together with transportation experts to discuss a wide variety of issues including: a new trolley system in Dania, obtaining funding/grants for transportation improvements, bus route improvements, a summit to educate the public on mass transportation, bus pass distribution, and providing transportation to nutrition sites (Meals on Wheels) for eligible seniors.   *continued*

FIGURE 6-1: CONTINUED

F. Children's Eligibility Initiatives

Initiated a program to help every eligible child in South Broward County to receive health insurance through the Florida KidCare Program which includes Medicaid, Medikids, and Healthy Kids. The effort to enroll these children includes door-to-door visits in underserved communities as well as enrollment sessions in local parks and community centers.

G. Adolescent Behavioral Health Programs

Developed a variety of behavioral health programs for adolescents including: New Solutions Program (an intensive outpatient program for substance-abusing children), Therapeutic After-School Program Services (TAPS) (a program for severely emotionally disturbed adolescents), Prime Time (a program to prevent juvenile crime and drug abuse at Apollo Middle School), and a Steps Program (an adolescent outpatient program).

DEVELOPING AND WORKING STRONG SUPPORT NETWORKS IN THE COMMUNITY

Efforts to raise funds and other resources for community benefit can include several systematic mechanisms that provide influential community members opportunities to help. For example, in one leading site, a foundation was established with four spin-off support groups (each with its own targeted efforts), two councils (with different targets), and finally, a committee that determines the true priorities in the community. These large networks may appear difficult to manage, but the goodwill, the political will, and the resources they bring to the organization make the benefits far outweigh the costs.

Mission Hospital Regional Medical Center

Before the Sisters of St. Joseph's of Orange took over Mission Hospital Regional Medical Center in Mission Viejo, California, a foundation was started by the physician owners of Mission Hospital with the purpose of providing community benefit. The Sisters decided to shift support to the hospital and transform the foundation into a control foundation—whose role is to support the hospital's need for philanthropy, including community programs. In fact, the community health programs affect all of the foundation's activities. Winnie Johnson, the foundation's president, has a board of 27 members and has been with the foundation for three and a half years.

Ms. Johnson thinks the foundation can be viewed as a model for quick adaptation to new directions. All the dollars raised come from members of the community, including corporations, employees, physicians, and other individuals. Fundraising efforts are extremely successful; recently the foundation received a $1.5 million gift, and raised $3.5 million in its first capital campaign. Now the foundation is completing its second capital campaign for $1.6 million.

But more than bricks and mortar are involved. Ms. Johnson is repeatedly told by community leaders and donors that the hospital's community programs have motivated their giving. The foundation has organized several groups to support its efforts, including the CEO's Advisory Council and the Women's Advisory Council.

CEO's Advisory Council   The CEO's Advisory Council meets quarterly with about 30 attendees of 50 total members. The members are community leaders, and the purpose of the council is to make the leaders aware of MHRMC's programs and to obtain their input. The chair of the board of the hospital serves as a member of this council as well. One or two foundation board members serve as members of the council, one of whom recruits other potential members to the council. Indeed, the council is used as a farm team to develop relationships and to recruit to the foundation board.

The purpose of the council is to communicate, and members are not solicited for contributions. Peter Bastone, the CEO, gives updates at each meeting, and a standing agenda item is advocacy updates—making the members aware of issues with the state and county in regard to children and patient rights, and so forth. Sometimes a member of the council will communicate back to the CEO relative to some proposed activity, and this kind of feedback has resulted in the appointment of a council member to the board of the hospital.

Women's Advisory Council   Winnie Johnson, president of the foundation, staffs the Women's Advisory Council, which meets quarterly and addresses women's issues—not labor, delivery, and menopause, but rather, how to deal with children, businesses, and eldercare. Leading women of the community are approached to serve. One member owns the largest property management agency in the county. She discussed property development in her area and how that might influence healthcare. Eventually she will spend some time with Peter Bastone (and make a contribution). This council has been very successful.

Support Groups The foundation board has four support groups—each with a cause. The foundation board members all serve on one of the support groups:

1. Camino Health Center: The center was founded to provide primary healthcare, dental care, and women's and infants' care (WIC) for indigent people. The foundation is instrumental in providing both financial and clinical support for the clinic. To provide dental care, for example, the foundation raises money and obtains service donations from dentists. Because the majority of the patients served come from the Latino community, the foundation is working to improve its relations and connections within that community. The foundation is helping to organize the leaders in the Latino community so that the foundation and community can "learn from each other." Over the next three to five years, Ms. Johnson will be asking the Latino community to help support a move to a more accessible location.

2. Thrift shop: The thrift shop provides an economical source of goods and supports Camino Health Center. Its role is to teach residents about ways to obtain free (MediCal) healthcare. The 65 volunteers and one paid manager are all aware of the values of Mission Hospital.

3. Grant proposals: One board support group is responsible to author grant proposals for the Camino Health Center, the Family Resource Center, asthma education, and so forth. Its job is to develop programs and services that donors want to support (which may not coincide with what the hospital or other caregivers most desperately think they need).

4. Valiant women—The board support group formed under the valiant women banner and comprised of philanthropic women from the community raises funds and provides educational experiences for donors or prospective donors on health, including financial health, women's health, mental health, and so forth.

Community Benefits Committee The community benefits committee is staffed by the vice president of mission and chaired by a member of the hospital board; the committee includes some physicians, but is mostly composed of community members. This committee determines the true priorities in the community and is driven by a community needs assessment. The Camino Health Center gets the majority of the Community Benefits Committee funds. Resources on conducting a community needs assessment are available from the Coalition for Healthy Cities and Communities (www.healthycommunities.org).

LESSONS LEARNED FROM THE DEMONSTRATION SITES

Marie Parham Hospital

Marie Parham Hospital in Henderson, North Carolina, has successfully developed ties to various groups in the community to provide for care to those without access through programs known as Healthy Access and the Four County Health Network (FCHN). Healthy Access operates through FCHN to serve the uninsured. FCHN offers better quality and low cost access through a network of primary care physicians in Granville and Vance counties. Conceived in 1996, FCHN coordinates the services of 51 physicians in its IPA, two hospitals in the four counties, as well as the Duke University and University of North Carolina medical centers. FCHN enables coordination with 1,500 physicians network wide, and with the public health services available in the area.

FCHN won its first direct contract in 1998, and then began more aggressively to seek contracts with self-insured employers. During 2000, several new direct contracts were entered including Paxton Media Group, publisher of the Daily Dispatch, with 100 covered lives, Ideal Fasteners with 400 covered lives, and Pacific Coast Bedding with 800 covered lives in the area.

The Duke Endowment and the Kate B. Reynolds Foundation have provided grants to FCHN to enable Healthy Access, starting on January 1, 2001. Healthy Access is an evolving patchwork quilt of services for the uninsured. The current grants, for example, underwrite subsidized prescriptions, capped at $750 per individual, and Patients In Need (PIN) home visits for benefits explanation. The Board of Directors decided that it would be financially prudent to conduct a pilot project for Healthy Access to assess the impact of the program prior to initiating the entire project. The pilot will incude 100 Vance County uninsured enrollees for a six-month period with an assessment of the project's value before instituting the full program.

CHAPTER SEVEN

Developing Processes that Promote Community Health

R EALLY A RESIDUAL strategy, processes that enhance community health are creative and useful practices that supplement the other strategies listed previously. Included in the following list are the CEO calendar audit and ways to improve the process of governance. Such processes are reminiscent of the continuous quality improvement initiatives that have improved hospital functioning in the past decade. We expect that additional processes will be added to this listing in the future as hospital leaders begin to introduce additional practices that fit their circumstances.

CONDUCTING CEO CALENDAR AUDITS OF COMMUNITY HEALTH ACTIVITIES

Either the CEO or the CEO and the board can establish an approximate percentage of time that the CEO should devote to community health. The CEO can then review his appointments over a period of time to determine if community health and other goals have received the appropriate levels of attention. This quick and simple method can help keep a busy executive on track.

Memorial Hospital and Health System

Many difficult challenges compete for a health system executive's time and effort. The CEO of Memorial Hospital and Health System in South Bend, Indiana, conducts periodic calendar audits to monitor and adjust how his time is allocated. Since the board and the CEO have determined that 25 to 30 percent of his time should be focused on community health initiatives, he expects this to be evident when he reviews his appointments. He keeps a complete log of his appointments. Looking back over his appointments from time to time lets him estimate how much time he spent on community health, as well as the other major goals of the organization.

HAVING AN ONGOING BOARD IMPROVEMENT PROCESS

The board improvement process, often initiated at a board retreat, is sustained by having a staff member of the hospital/system who is trained in group process and decision making provide feedback to the chairman after each board meeting. The purpose of the feedback is to ensure broad participation and sufficient discussion of issues. One of the trained staff person's roles in this capacity is to demonstrate to the chair and CEO how well-balanced the organization's attention to its various goals has been in each meeting.

Cambridge Health Alliance

The Cambridge Health Alliance parent board in Cambridge, Massachusetts, conducts monthly meetings with a set two-hour agenda. The first hour is typically occupied by the review of a consent agenda and presentation and discussion of major strategic issues requested by the board. During the latter half of the meeting, the CEO presents an administrative update on the state of the organization and its performance. This segment is often interactive and takes up one-quarter of the entire meeting. The final 30-minute segment of the parent board's meeting focuses on board self-evaluation and improvement.

The board self-evaluation and improvement is an unfinished process that was initiated first in 1994 when a prominent physician expert in the area of performance improvement was recruited by the CEO to join the executive team. A board retreat in March 1997 focused on the board improvement process with special attention to the board's role in the community. The other chief roles emerging from this board self-improvement process were mission definition, high-level policy setting, and monitoring performance against policy.

Perhaps the most unusual practice that was established at the board retreat was providing the chairman with personal one-on-one feedback on his performance in chairing the board. The current vice president for organizational development was invited to a board meeting, and when she gave a few reactions to the chairing of the meeting, the chairman requested that she continue this practice to improve his leadership with the board.

Typical feedback includes how the chairman could include more members in the discussion, how debate can be furthered, and how issues can be more completely explored. The practice of ongoing process improvement is evident; in this case, the emphasis is on how board meetings are conducted. Obviously, this kind of feedback can only succeed with a secure board chairman and a skilled and tactful counselor.

Although the composition of the parent board is fixed by the enabling legislation that created the public authority, the county's Joint Public Health Board is undergoing its own improvement process. Established to ensure coordination on community health efforts across the two cities, the Joint Public Health Board is aggressively revisiting its composition.

The Joint Public Health Board has focused its energy on ensuring that it reflects the diversity of the community it serves. It has been largely successful through the use of such interesting approaches as advertising the availability of board positions in two major weeklies in Cambridge and Somerville and on the radio. However, the board continues to lack participation from certain linguistic minorities who make up a large portion of the community's population.

To achieve better diversity and retain an appropriately skilled and capable board, all current members were asked to sign a tender of resignation. Each was also asked to indicate whether they would seek another one-, two-, or three-year term or would prefer to resign from the board but continue to volunteer in some other capacity. In the context of a series of discussions about the need for the board to improve itself, in part by better reflecting the composition of the community, this approach is expected to accelerate progress in achieving the board's goals in composition, as well as create opportunities to recruit "new talent." Several members have left the board as a result of this reorganization but will continue to contribute in other volunteer capacities. More importantly, representatives of the Hispanic, Haitian-American, and Portuguese-speaking communities are now better represented on the board.

LESSONS LEARNED FROM THE DEMONSTRATION SITES

Evergreen Community Health Care

Evergreen Community Health Care in Kirkland, Washington, has adopted several new practices to achieve better community health and keep board members better informed about the status of community health initiatives. Board members receive a quarterly report on the use of the levy funds, including systematic investments in community health initiatives. These reports help board members communicate consistently and clearly with other community groups. Also, management provides board members and others with standard PowerPoint presentation packages for use in public speaking settings. ECHC is initiating an annual retreat to discuss community health status with executives, medical staff, and the board.

St. Joseph Healthcare

St. Joseph Healthcare in Albuquerque, New Mexico, developed a new board self-evaluation process. SJH formed a three-member team to initiate the project, including the vice president responsible for mission services, the vice president for organizational development and human resources, and a member of the board. The team made a few recommendations that addressed the goal of developing a comprehensive board evaluation process. Specifically it recommended that the first half-hour of every board meeting be devoted to an educational session to include a focus on mission and healthy community issues. The board should also receive a written summary report from the quality and mission committee. In addition, the board was advised to conduct an annual self-assessment that includes community health as a criterion. Finally, a community health assessment would be presented to the board on an annual basis.

St. Joseph found that not every board meeting could incorporate an educational session. A board self-assessment was developed with one of the four principal sections entitled, "Mission and Values." The new instrument was well received by the board.

Texas Health Resources

Texas Health Resources in Irving, Texas, added a section to their board's self-assessment titled, "Community Health and Benefit Oversight." The executive vice president of corporate affairs stated that a survey of trustees was conducted on the needs of their communities. Although the survey focused more on finance and quality, it also touched on the board's responsibility for and oversight of community health. The VP felt that a newsletter might help achieve a serious review of community health.

Kaleida Health

Kaleida Health in Buffalo, New York, also effected a board self-assessment in order to monitor the community health involvement of the board. Figure 7-1 contains the questions asked of the board; the confidential responses were combined and results were reported at the following board retreat.

CHANNELING MARKETING COSTS OF COMPETITORS TO BENEFIT THE COMMUNITY

A healthcare provider with strong community relations and customer loyalty can take a leadership role in creating collaboration where large outside managed care companies might otherwise fragment and disrupt the delivery system through competition. A local CEO might pledge to negotiate with the competitors in an even-handed way and encourage the allocation of capitated lives based on preexisting physician loyalties. As a result, marketing battle costs can be diverted to a synergistic end, such as developing a health institute to examine clinical and community health practices.

FIGURE 7-1: KALEIDA HEALTH BOARD OF DIRECTORS
SELF-ASSESSMENT SURVEY

Part A: **OPEN-ENDED QUESTIONS**

1. Of the things the Board has done during the past year, what one or two do you feel were most successful?

2. Are there shortcomings in the Board's organization or performance that need attention? If yes, please describe.

Part B: **BOARD REPORT CARD (1999–2000 Board Year)**

Instructions

Kaleida has dealt with a number of important issues this year. On the next page is a list of some very important ones. If we have not included an issue you think should be on the list, there is a place to add it.

Please consider the work that the board has done on each issue. Based on the level of involvement appropriate for a board, assign a grade _**for our work as a board.**_ Use the following grading system:

Grading System for Board Report Card

A =   We addressed this issue in a high-quality and timely fashion.
      I feel good, I feel proud.

B =   We addressed it, but some aspects could have been improved.
      Generally, not bad!

C =   We discussed this, but I am not satisfied with our performance on this item.
      We should have handled this better.

D/F = Our actions were inadequate or we did not address the issue.
       Very poor performance.

continued

FIGURE 7-1: CONTINUED

Kaleida Health Board Report Card (1999–2000 Board Year)

ISSUE	GRADE	COMMENTS (explain if "C" or "D/F")
1. Fiscal Responsibility		
2. Community Health		
3. Educational Affiliations with University of Buffalo		
4. Strategic Plan Roll-Out		
5A. Master Facilities Plan: Children's Hospital		
5B. Master Facilities Plan: Millard Suburban Hosp.		
5C. Master Facilities Plan: Other Facilities		
6. Clinical Service Line Development		
7. Quality/Service Excellence		
8. Info Systems—Y2K		
9. Management Performance Assessment		
10. Medical Staff Oversight		
11. Employee Workforce Oversight		
12. Other:		

Part C:	THE WORK OF THE BOARD

Answer the questions listed below by checking the response that most closely represents your view:

1. Our board monitors and evaluates proposals brought before the board, including initiatives of subsidiary organizations, to ensure they are consistent with our system's mission, vision, and values.

_____ Strongly Disagree   _____ Disagree   _____ Agree   _____ Strongly Agree

continued

2. Our board members are active and effective in representing the community's healthcare interests and serve as a communication link between the hospital, government officials, and others important to the provision of health services.

___ Strongly Disagree ___ Disagree ___ Agree ___ Strongly Agree

3. The board ensures that perspectives and issues from the appropriate constituencies are addressed in the planning process.

___ Strongly Disagree ___ Disagree ___ Agree ___ Strongly Agree

4. The board recognizes how quality of services must be closely related to our strategic planning and budgeting oversight responsibilities.

___ Strongly Disagree ___ Disagree ___ Agree ___ Strongly Agree

5. The information the board receives about the quality of care and the quality improvement program is complete and adequate for board-level discussion and decision making.

___ Strongly Disagree ___ Disagree ___ Agree ___ Strongly Agree

6. We regularly assess and can readily demonstrate that our organization provides a high level of benefit to our community.

___ Strongly Disagree ___ Disagree ___ Agree ___ Strongly Agree

7. The board is providing effective leadership in monitoring organizational performance to ensure our commitment to quality.

___ Strongly Disagree ___ Disagree ___ Agree ___ Strongly Agree

8. We approve and monitor the progress of financial policies, plans, programs, and standards to ensure preservation and enhancement of the system's financial assets and resources.

___ Strongly Disagree ___ Disagree ___ Agree ___ Strongly Agree

9. The board receives financial reports in a format conducive to its analysis/understanding.

___ Strongly Disagree ___ Disagree ___ Agree ___ Strongly Agree

10. There is a positive relationship between the board and the senior management team (including physicians).

___ Strongly Disagree ___ Disagree ___ Agree ___ Strongly Agree

11. I am satisfied with the effectiveness of the board's agenda.

___ Strongly Disagree ___ Disagree ___ Agree ___ Strongly Agree

12. The frequency and duration of board and committee meetings are adequate to conduct the board's oversight responsibilities, but do not discourage attendance and participation by misusing valuable trustee time.

___ Strongly Disagree ___ Disagree ___ Agree ___ Strongly Agree

continued

FIGURE 7-1: CONTINUED

13. The board chair exercises appropriate leadership to ensure that all board members have equal opportunity to participate and agenda items are dispatched after reasonable discussion.

___ Strongly Disagree   ___ Disagree   ___ Agree   ___ Strongly Agree

14. The information the board receives from management is complete and adequate for board-level discussion and decision making.

___ Strongly Disagree   ___ Disagree   ___ Agree   ___ Strongly Agree

15. We have adequate informal/social opportunities to get to know fellow board members.

___ None   ___ Too Few   ___ Enough   ___ Too Many

Part D: INDIVIDUAL SELF-ASSESSMENT

16. As regards knowledge about the current healthcare environment, I rate myself as:

___ 1 Not at all knowledgeable about healthcare

___ 2 Somewhat knowledgeable

___ 3 Adequately knowledgeable for board membership

___ 4 Quite knowledgeable

___ 5 An expert on the healthcare environment

17. Using the categories below, describe the way time for speaking in a board meeting is used by members of this board. (Please distribute 100 percentage points.)

A ___ % of members talk more than they need to (to make their point)

B ___ % of members take about their fair share of the time

C ___ % of members wish to say more, but do not

D ___ % of members say almost nothing at most meetings

E ___ % of members _____
                                    (optional fill in)
100 %

18. Using the categories listed above, I see myself most of the time in category:

___ A ___ B ___ C ___ D ___ E (check one)

19. Using the categories listed above, I think most other people on the board probably see me in category:

___ A ___ B ___ C ___ D ___ E (check one)

continued

20. On this board: (circle one)

It's hard to get
a word in and say   1   2   3   4   5   I have no trouble
what I am thinking   getting people's
                                                            full attention

21. I am a member of the _____ board committee.

The time I spend at meetings of this committee is: (circle one)

Very unproductive;   1   2   3   4   5   A very productive
A waste of time   use of time

22. I am also a member of the _____ board committee.

The time I spend at meetings of this committee is: (circle one)

Very unproductive;   1   2   3   4   5   A very productive
A waste of time   use of time

23. To what extent do you feel you are making a significant contribution
through your membership on this board? (circle one)

Not at all   1   2   3   4   5   A great deal

24. To what extent do you feel you are doing your share as a board member?
(circle one)

Doing less than   1   2   3   4   5   Doing more than
my share   my share

25. I think the most important thing the board should be working on next year
for Kaleida's future success is:

Cambridge Health Alliance

Recently, Cambridge Health Alliance confronted a major issue when the system contemplated allying with one of two large, competing vertically integrated systems. Partners, the system that owns Massachusetts General Hospital and the Brigham and Women's hospitals, had the allegiance of about two-thirds of the Cambridge and Somerville physicians. Caregroup, the other system that owns the neighboring Mt. Auburn Hospital, is strongly affiliated with about one-third of the Alliance's physicians.

The CEO was reluctant to align his organization exclusively with either system, knowing that it would inevitably affect the collaborative relationships that Cambridge had with both systems. He persuaded both systems to affiliate with Cambridge and agreed to build a firewall between administrators and physicians at Cambridge who are responsible to each system so as to protect confidentiality and ensure compliance with anti-trust regulations.

This exceptional "no-fly zone" was accomplished because both systems recognized that the Alliance is committed to the entire community's well-being and plays a unique role as a safety net provider. The arrangement also enabled Cambridge to preserve its existing referral networks to other area hospitals.

An additional benefit of this arrangement is that the three organizations agreed to jointly fund an Institute for Community Health that will conduct research on effective clinical and community health programs using the expertise of the researchers from all three systems and researchers at Harvard University.

CHAPTER EIGHT

Conclusion

A MERICA'S HOSPITALS LEAD the world in advanced medicine. This leadership stems from a major investment of resources, incredible scientific advances, and intricate organizational arrangements that permit the delivery of coordinated, comprehensive medical care. In spite of the miracles worked every day, people often do not love their hospitals and sometimes distrust them outright. The highly trained personnel who work miracles in hospitals usually feel the same way. Hospitals have been unable to generate the sustained flow of goodwill and support that they might deserve. To the people who make them work, the general public, and public officials, hospitals often seem to be driven by their assets, competitive plans, and strategic business models.

This image constrains hospitals from capturing the hearts as well as the minds of community members, staff, and others. The great potential of knowledgeable customers, loyal staff, and committed community partners is left undiscovered or underused in many communities, weakening hospitals financially and politically. Even more important over the long term, these underused connections make it impossible, unlikely, or more difficult than necessary to exploit modern knowledge about health education, disease prevention, early diagnosis, and other approaches to fostering health in the community.

Today especially, hospital executives and boards feel pressure to maintain the organization's financial solvency, as insurers and the government reduce payments to them. Hospitals do face tremendous challenges. But concentrating only against the most apparent enemy and pushing against that one force, pulls attention away from other sources of strength and other pieces of information in the environment. Increasing the hospital's emphasis on community health can provide strength and information that will help the hospital leadership meets its goals.

Your community provides customers, staff, and partners. Intelligence about your community, and its diversity, can improve service design and delivery. Organizing better around community health goals can produce higher quality and lower costs. Advancing community health can be a source of personal and professional satisfaction, adding balance to your life and reducing the risk of burnout. Members of your community can be political advocates. In these and other ways, attending more to community health can benefit the people in your area, as your mission guides you to do. Your efforts in the community can, and should, simultaneously benefit the hospital as it strives toward excellence in meeting its mission and goals. The secret to overcoming the tremendous challenges of hospital leadership lies both in operational efficiencies and in a community health ethic.

In this book, executives and board members from leading hospitals offer organizational practices that you can use to better organize your hospital's management and governance around community health. Few of the practices we have documented are new. All of them have been used in the real world. At least one hospital or health system sees each practice as providing greater benefits than costs. We sought to provide a cafeteria of practices that could be described well enough so you could consider them all and adopt one or a few that make the most sense to you.

The practices documented in this book are not community health interventions, such as can be found today in virtually every community. Instead, the practices we discuss are meant specifically for hospital and health system leadership, and they are about how to run a hospital or system. Adopting them can increase expectations about community health within the organization. Building these practices into the routine management and governance of the hospital or health system will contribute to a shift in the organization's culture. Taken collectively, these practices describe a rich set of behaviors that one would find only in a hospital or health system that had developed a culture in which community health is as important as financial performance. We believe that an internal culture like this will express itself in superior performance in many ways, including ways that are most evident outside the hospital itself.

INITIATING STRATEGIES TO MOTIVATE INVOLVEMENT IN COMMUNITY HEALTH

We have identified seven strategies that leading hospitals use to motivate their involvement in community health activities, and within each strategy cataloged a number of specific practices. Here are some ideas that you might want to think about in deciding how your hospital should proceed to implement some of these practices.

The Visioning Strategy

The board and management have an opportunity to affect how the hospital relates to its community service mission by reviewing the existing mission statement and making the modifications needed to assert the importance of this goal. Prime opportunities to recraft the statement exist in mergers and consolidations, but this is also desirable when initiating a new strategic plan. Goals, set out each year, also need to include something about community health.

Our demonstration sites taught us something about implementing goals into the hospital's visioning strategy. For example, St. Mary Medical Center quite easily added its community health objectives to its two-page dashboard that guides board discussion at every meeting. This enabled SMMC to evaluate multiple bottom lines, just as Citrus Valley Health Partners suggested. Likewise, Kaleida Health has incorporated community health as a top-level goal in its strategic plan.

Texas Health Resources apparently encountered a few difficulties in establishing community health as a system goal and as an agenda item at every system board meeting. Moreover, even though all of its affiliated hospitals have adopted the current system's goal to prevent family violence, it has proved more difficult to incorporate general community health issues on every hospital board agenda.

Similarly, while the subcommittee of the quality and mission committee of St. Joseph Healthcare in Albuquerque recommended that the first half hour of every board meeting be devoted to an educational session to include a focus on mission and healthy community issues, the urgency of their current fiscal crisis precluded this from happening. Thus, visioning and goal setting, while relatively low-cost efforts, can sometimes be held up because of reluctance to change or because of other pressing events. Perhaps the best advice we can offer is to be persistent and try to incorporate visioning practices in times of relatively less turmoil.

The Financing Strategy

Today great variation exists among hospitals' financial success. For hospitals with positive operating margins, leaders are advised to consider systematically funding programs that promote community health. For those with negative operating margins, leaders may wish to consider tying executive compensation to at least one community health objective. In effect, we recommend that some practice within this strategy should be considered by all hospitals, because it shows commitment in a tangible way and motivates behaviors that cannot be ignored inside or outside the hospital.

Through our demonstration sites' efforts to incorporate some leading financial practices, we learned that some were immediately applicable. For example, Memorial Hospital and Health System's tithe-o-meter was used by Evergreen Community Health Care in selecting its grant recipients. Moreover, like Memorial, ECHC appointed a manager to oversee the grants and open roadblocks that might get in the way of sponsored partners.

We also learned that Memorial Hospital and Health System's grassroots approach to funding partners could be modified and still result in apparently constructive programs. Specifically, Evergreen Community Health Care decided to target specific populations that would be beneficiaries of their awards. By focusing on the elderly who lack access to care, the disabled elderly, and children with asthma, ECHC awarded fewer but larger grants and thus assured themselves that their funding would have a sizeable effect.

One system tried but failed to begin to systematically tithe. Texas Health Resources had the best intentions but, because of its focus on an unrealized merger with Baylor Health System, the time, attention, and resources needed to institute tithing were not forthcoming during the year of study. In our final interviews, system executives and board members said they were considering various strategies to systematically fund community health initiatives—like reducing corporate overhead to allow hospitals to fund community health projects locally. Also, the system's foundations were considering ways to raise money to effect this objective. The important point in this situation is that systematic funding is *now* on THR's radar screen.

The Education Strategy

The education strategy proposes a solution to reawaken board members', hospital managers', and staff members' understanding of the purpose of hospitals in society. By initiating community plunges, linking with universities and other centers of creativity, and systematizing the education of new staff, hospitals will develop the human resource reservoir that motivates desired behaviors. Thus, recrafting a mission statement needs to be followed by teaching the mission and showing with real community examples how the organization can materially improve community health.

Our demonstration sites offer some guidance on how education for boards and managers can be structured and what obstacles might need to be overcome. For example, Evergreen Community Health Center began a program to jointly educate the board, senior managers, and members of the medical staff using local university talent. We learned that some logistical issues presented relative to getting good attendance; few medical staff were able to attend the first of several planned sessions. Moreover, the topic for training was selected by the leadership rather than by representatives of those who would be attending. Despite this, one unanticipated conse-quence was improved relationships with the medical school officials who reportedly were delighted to be called on to facilitate the learning. Over time, we might anticipate that joint education will foster more common understandings of community health problems and their solutions.

The Personnel Strategy

The traditional role of vice presidents in charge of relating to external agen-cies has been based on a marketing or public relations purpose. Practices promoted in the personnel strategy suggest that a special high-level posi-tion be established, reporting directly to the CEO, that focuses some of the time on developing partnerships that advance community health. Other practices integrate the evaluation of boards and executives to form a re-inforcing system that emphasizes the importance of goals promoting com-munity health. These and other practices show how individuals can modify their routine behaviors to advance the hospital's mission and their own self-actualization.

What have our demonstration sites taught us? We evidenced some suc-cesses but also some mixed successes and failures in hospitals' efforts to incorporate personnel practices promoting community health. While Maria Parham Hospital in Henderson, North Carolina, intended to make community health an explicit part of its board's work, this element of its work plan was not accomplished. The community health needs in this small community, board members asserted, were recognizable to the board, and they felt that needs would bubble up as issues demanded resolution. Part of the failure may rest on the fact that the CEO who had committed to this practice was replaced during the study period.

Texas Health Resources reported that its boards' self-evaluation now in-cluded community health as a criterion. But one executive we interviewed suggested that some education of local hospital boards might be a good idea—to ensure that they focus on legitimate community health issues as opposed to clinical issues. This executive suggested that a newsletter to teach board members about community outreach might be needed.

THR was able to revise its managers' evaluations to include community health as a criterion—both in respect to individual evaluations and in their 360-degree evaluations. One interesting innovation was the possible incor-poration of a new position to be developed that would focus on community health evaluation. The purpose of this position would be to show the hos-pitals the business benefits that derive from community health efforts.

Two sites were successful in revising their board self-evaluations—Kaleida Health was especially successful in that an industrial psychologist was employed to develop a valid instrument. St. Joseph Healthcare also revised its board's self-evaluation. Evaluations can be revised with a champion, but we also observed that the actual criteria developed for assessment may need to be explained to ensure that evaluations are understood by each board member and manager involved.

The Marketing Strategy

If personnel practices focus on modifying individual behaviors, marketing practices consider the hospital's initiatives as an organization. Hospitals need to listen to the voices in their community. Community needs can be discerned scientifically, and some hospitals have incorporated creative ways to tap community leaders' perceptions of the most needed programs. At the other end of the spectrum, hospitals need to communicate with their communities about health status developments and issues, and they need to partner with others without necessarily demanding recognition for providing help.

This strategy was the one most often adopted by the demonstration sites. Nearly all sites planned and advanced their marketing efforts relative to community health, if for no other reason than to publicize their having been selected as a demonstration site. Perhaps the most ambitious effort to identify community health needs was Kaleida's Summit. This effort taught the value of giving the organizing credit to a common community benefit agency—the United Way. Also, holding the Summit at a site accessible to both rural and urban residents helped achieve buy-in from all groups.

Even Maria Parham Hospital, which experienced difficult financial problems during the study year, put out numerous reports to its community through the efforts of its marketing director. St. Mary Medical Center was able to build on its earlier success in establishing a community-wide forum to obtain "Well City Status" and initiated a Community Health Council with the mayor's help. Evergreen Community Health Care also collected data and issued an especially useful one-page summary of its community health initiatives to show where the public levy funds were being used. ECHC also created a PowerPoint presentation for its officials to use. Finally, Texas Health Resources used its community health councils to tell system officials about local community needs.

All of these examples show that listening and reporting back to the community can be achieved through ambitious undertakings. The key is to follow through on the listening part; already Kaleida has shown itself to be on the leading edge by forming various task forces. How this reporting out has enhanced the image of the demonstration sites is at this time unclear.

The Structures Strategy

As large organizations, hospitals have the opportunity to reach out to their communities systematically by organizing units and committees. If the purpose of a board committee is to analyze and report on quality and community outreach, then the chances are great that these issues will be discussed and attended to by the hospital. Similarly, if committees or councils are formed that draw in the views of diverse community members, then the hospital can be more certain that it will reach these segments of their constituency. The point is that units created with clear scope and function statements help to systematize a hospital's attention to community health.

Two demonstration site experiences aided our understanding of the issues involved in developing structures to support community health. First, Kaleida's board planning committee now routinely reports on community health progress to the full board, and Kaleida's comprehensive operating plan has grown from three objectives related to community health to seven. Thus, by charging an existing board committee with community health functions, the leadership of hospitals can monitor and grow its activities in this arena.

St. Mary Medical Center established a community health council, but it has only met once, and it is too soon to determine its effect on community health promotion. Creating a council of key players in the community requires a good deal of advance work, the support of political figures, and a facilitator to ensure that the agenda moves along.

The Processes Strategy

Just as structures form the architecture for ensuring that the hospital pay attention to community health, processes help systematize the CEO's and the board's work toward the same end. This is really a residual category—containing practices that could not easily be included in one of the six previously listed strategies. Over time, we can expect that creative hospital leaders will add to the menu of practices we have identified and described.

Leaders of hospitals need to craft a vision and identify structures and processes that can transform their organizations from inwardly directed medical delivery sites to outwardly directed proactive institutions bent on improving their community members' health. By opening themselves up to the possibilities of improved community heath, we know hospitals can and will rekindle the flame of a dedicated staff and an appreciative community.

Appendix
The Role of Public Health

This book about practices that hospitals can adopt to implement community health purposes would be incomplete without some mention of the role of local public health departments in the leading and demonstration sites. When we visited leading hospitals, we observed interesting differences in their relationships with public health agencies. For example, the CEO of the Cambridge Health Alliance is also the chief public health official of Somerville and Cambridge. In other sites such as Citrus Valley Health Partners and Memorial Healthcare System, close ties were evident between the hospitals and public health. In fact, the senior vice president for mission integration and community care at CVHP was being loaned to the county public health authority to assist it in implementing programs for community benefit. In still other leading sites, we saw no direct or even indirect involvement with public health agencies.

Our consultants recommended that we pay special attention to the demonstration sites' relationships with public health agencies in the area. Again, we observed a great deal of variation; relationships ranged from close integration and the provision of complementary services, to noncommunication and duplication of services. Examples of integrated and complementary relationships include Evergreen Community Health Care and Kaleida.

At Evergreen Community Health Care, the public health district director recognized the hospital as a strong partner and supporter of public and community health efforts. Some Evergreen personnel are former employees of the health department, and Evergreen always invites a public health presence to its events and educational seminars. The director considers Evergreen as a model for hospitals in their collaboration on community and public health issues.

At Kaleida Health, Erie County's commissioner of public health retired during the study year, but the new commissioner pointed out that in his view, the Summit had fostered greater collaboration among Kaleida, the competing Catholic system, and the public health agency. For example, the health department launched an insurance plan for those without health coverage, and he observed that the health department had been busier during the past year than before. The commissioner concluded that an umbrella group is needed to manage the process of coordinating the entire greater Buffalo community's health effort, now that silos have been broken down.

Somewhere between the extremes of integration and lack of communication between hospitals and their local departments of public health are Texas Health Resources, Maria Parham Hospital, and St. Joseph Healthcare. At Texas Health Resources, we visited with officials from the Fort Worth Department of Public Health. One of THR's teaching hospitals was providing a mobile prostate and breast screening unit that the city public health department would publicize at its health fairs. But public health is not rewarded for such collaboration, so structural problems need to be overcome to maximize such partnerships. Recently, an emergency preparedness team had been put into place with officials of municipal agencies and hospitals appointed to focus on various health issues. Now a metropolitan response system for emergencies has been established and special hotlines link the collaborators.

At Maria Parham Hospital, the public health department views itself as a direct ally of providers in Henderson, North Carolina. The department works to ensure quality of healthcare services rather than providing services directly. Increasing collaboration between the hospital and department was evident recently, as the department has been using the hospital's auditorium for health education. The hospital also established a clinic to serve referrals from the health department's STD discovery efforts. But overall, the county health officer observed that better coordination is needed between the public health department and local providers like Maria Parham Hospital.

In Albuquerque, St. Joseph Healthcare's relationship with the public health department is positive and productive. For example, the department is able to assist community coalitions by providing data as providers seek external funding. But poor funding for the local health department during the study year saw the abolition of its Healthier Communities unit, and despite authorization no new hiring has occurred because of lack of funding. Overall, the public health department has few resources to offer providers, and it is mostly through private sector collaborations that community health may be enhanced.

In Hobart, Indiana, St. Mary Medical Center executives told us that little interaction took place between the hospital and public health officials. We noted the seemingly redundant efforts to measure blood pressure and provide influenza immunizations. The public health administrator suggested that the department and the hospital might be more effective if they each targeted a unique segment of the community for such prevention programs. Recently, lead poisoning was identified as a major hazard; SMMC may be involved in screening while other federal agencies may be involved in correcting structural defects in homes. The department administrator felt that improved communication with SMMC would be beneficial, but hospital officials were skeptical that sufficient public health resources were available to significantly effect positive outcomes.

Efforts are underway to help ensure that public health agencies become more involved with and integrate services they provide with local hospitals and other health providers. As hospitals begin to reach out to their communities, they will likely be drawn to public health agencies that can serve as useful and instructive allies to improve community health.

Selected References

American College of Healthcare Executives. 2000 (revised). "Healthcare Executives' Responsibility to Their Communities." Public Policy Statement. ACHE (www.ache.org/policy/respon.html).

———. 1997. "The Healthcare Executive's Role in Community Health Improvement." Public Policy Statement. ACHE.

Bogue, R. J. 1999. "An Incentive for Community Health." *Trustee* 52 (5): 14–19.

Chyna, J. J. 2001. "Enhancing Your Public Image." *Healthcare Executive* 16 (1): 7–11.

Milstead, L. 1999. "The Pressure Is On: Tying Executive Pay to Community Benefits." *Health Forum Journal* 42 (2): 47–49.

Nelson, J. C., H. Rashid, V. G. Galvin, J. D. Essien, and L. M. Levine. 1999. "Public/Private Partners: Key Factors in Creating a Strategic Alliance for Community Health." *American Journal of Preventive Medicine* 16 (3, Suppl.): 94–102.

Proenca, E. J. 1998. "Community Orientation in Health Services Organizations: The Concept and Its Implementation." *Health Care Management Review* 23 (2): 28–38.

Smith, T. 1996. "Urban Hospitals Use Community, Business Ties to Improve Public Health, Reduce Violence." *Healthcare Strategic Management* 14 (8): 16–17.

Weil, P. A., and R. J. Bogue. 1999. "Providing Community Health Services: Leading Practices You Can Use." *Healthcare Executive* 14 (6): 18–24.

About the Authors

Peter A. Weil, Ph.D., FACHE

Dr. Peter A. Weil is vice president of the division of research and development of the American College of Healthcare Executives. In addition to leading the current study of hospital management and governance practices that promote community health, he conducts periodic surveys to compare executives' careers by gender and race/ethnicity. He also conducts market research to assess members' interest and satisfaction with the ACHE's programs and services.

Prior to joining ACHE in 1982, Dr. Weil was the director of the National Study of Internal Medicine Manpower based at the University of Chicago; he also taught social epidemiology in the graduate program in hospital and health administration at the University of Chicago.

He has served on the board of the healthcare division of the Academy of Management and The Selfhelp Home, a retirement and skilled nursing facility for refugees from Nazi Germany. He received his master's degree in health administration from the University of Iowa and his doctorate in medical sociology from the University of Chicago.

Richard J. Bogue, Ph.D.

After serving in the Air Force, Dr. Richard J. Bogue received his doctorate in human communication and taught intercultural, political, organizational, and interpersonal communication at the University of South Florida, la Universidad de las Americas (Mexico), the University of Texas, and the University of Illinois at Chicago. He also has taught health policy and politics at Governors State University. Dr. Bogue joined the American Hospital Association's Health Research and Educational Trust in 1988. At the Trust, Dr. Bogue led a series of demonstration and research projects, most on the theme of community-responsive health system improvement. In 1997, Dr. Bogue became senior director of governance programs with the AHA's Division of Trustee and Community Leadership, where he produced a series of educational programs and publications for healthcare leaders.

Dr. Bogue now runs Richard Bogue and Affiliates, a consultant group focusing on improving governance and community partnerships. He currently has formal affiliations with Kailo Alliance, which develops rural community health plans, and Health System Synergies, which helps health systems discover collaborative synergies amidst their competitive challenges.

Dr. Bogue is board chair for Henry Booth House, a nonprofit social service agency on Chicago's south side. He has authored several books, including *Health Care for the 21st Century: Community-Oriented Primary Care* and *Health Network Innovations: How 20 Communities Are Improving Their Systems Through Collaboration.*

Reed L. Morton, Ph.D., FACHE

Dr. Reed L. Morton is director of the Healthcare Executive Career Resource Center at the American College of Healthcare Executives. Dr. Morton's healthcare career has been multifaceted. It includes teaching and administrative appointments at the Universities of Iowa, Michigan, Chicago, and Notre Dame. He has directed health planning with public agencies and private health systems. Dr. Morton joined the staff of the American College of Healthcare Executives in 1987 to head the Hospital Leadership Project. Subsequent assignments included coordinating the Carolinas Healthcare Leadership Demonstration Project and several task forces on career development. He has authored articles on healthcare marketing, governance and leadership, and career development. He is a past president of the Chicago Health Executives Forum and served on the boards of the healthcare division of the Academy of Management and the Administrative Fellowship Coordinating Council. He is a member of the International Association of Career Management Professionals and serves as a reviewer for such journals as Medical Care and Health Care Management Review.

Practical Governance
J. Larry Tyler, FACHE, FAAHC, and Errol L. Biggs, Ph.D., FACHE

This quick read is the perfect tool for board member training or getting your board back on track. It covers the basics of governance from board structure and board education to CEO selection and crisis management. Useful tools including sample job descriptions, a sample board meeting agenda, and a board self-assessment tool can be adapted and used at your organization right away.

"Practical Governance is certainly the best discussion of hospital governance issues that I have encountered .... I am obtaining a copy for each of my own board members and also my senior staff."

—Deryl E. Gulliford, CEO, Stevens County Hospital, Kansas

Order No. BKCO-1116, $50
Softbound, 198 pp, 2001, ISBN 1-56793-147-2
An ACHE Management Series Book

Who Will Pay for Long Term Care?
Insights from the Partnership Programs
Edited by Nelda McCall

Thirty-nine percent of the population over 65 will spend at least some time in a nursing home before they die. However, few people have stopped to think about how they would pay for such care. This book explores the significant challenge of long term care financing. It includes expert commentary on the early successes and failures of the Partnership for Long Term Care, an effort funded by The Robert Wood Johnson Foundation that encouraged cooperation between public and private sectors. The book offers insights about the politics of healthcare financing, the workings of the insurance market, and the process of state health financing reform.

Order No. BKCO-1123, $52
Softbound, 331 pp, August 2001, ISBN 1-56793-097-2
An Academy/HAP Book

Prices do not include shipping and are subject to change.
To order, call (301) 362-6905 or order online at www.ache.org/hap.html